EAT RIGHT
FOR
YOUR
INFLAMMATION
TYPE

EAT RIGHT
FOR
YOUR
INFLAMMATION
TYPE

**The Three-Step Program to
Strengthen Immunity, Heal Chronic
Pain, and Boost Your Energy**

MAGGIE BERGHOFF, FNP-C

ATRIA BOOKS

NEW YORK   LONDON   TORONTO   SYDNEY   NEW DELHI

ATRIA
BOOKS

An Imprint of Simon & Schuster, Inc.
1230 Avenue of the Americas
New York, NY 10020

First Atria Books hardcover edition December 2021

ATRIA B O O K S and colophon are trademarks of Simon & Schuster, Inc.

For information about special discounts for bulk purchases, please contact Simon & Schuster Special Sales at 1-866-506-1949 or business@simonandschuster.com.

The Simon & Schuster Speakers Bureau can bring authors to your live event. For more information or to book an event, contact the Simon & Schuster Speakers Bureau at 1-866-248-3049 or visit our website at www.simonspeakers.com.

Interior design by Timothy Shaner, NightandDayDesign.biz

Manufactured in the United States of America

1 3 5 7 9 10 8 6 4 2

Library of Congress Cataloging-in-Publication Data

Names: Berghoff, Maggie, author.
Title: Eat right for your inflammation type : the three-step program to strengthen immunity, heal chronic pain, and boost your energy / Maggie Berghoff, FNP-C.
Description: First Atria books hardcover edition. | New York : Atria Books, 2021. | Includes bibliographical references and index.
Identifiers: LCCN 2021042800 (print) | LCCN 2021042801 (ebook) | ISBN 9781982157647 (hardcover) | ISBN 9781982157661 (ebook)
Subjects: LCSH: Inflammation—Popular works. | Inflammation—Diet Therapy—Popular works. | Nutrition—Popular works. | Self-care, Health—Popular works.
Classification: LCC RB131 .B47 2021 (print) | LCC RB131 (ebook) | DDC 616/.0473—dc23
LC record available at https://lccn.loc.gov/2021042800
LC ebook record available at https://lccn.loc.gov/2021042801

ISBN 978-1-9821-5764-7
ISBN 978-1-9821-5766-1 (ebook)

To my family, I love you with all my heart and am so incredibly grateful.

To you, as you pick up this book, may it impact you and everyone around you in the most positive way.

CONTENTS

STEP THREE

EAT TO TREAT

EAT RIGHT
FOR
YOUR
INFLAMMATION
TYPE

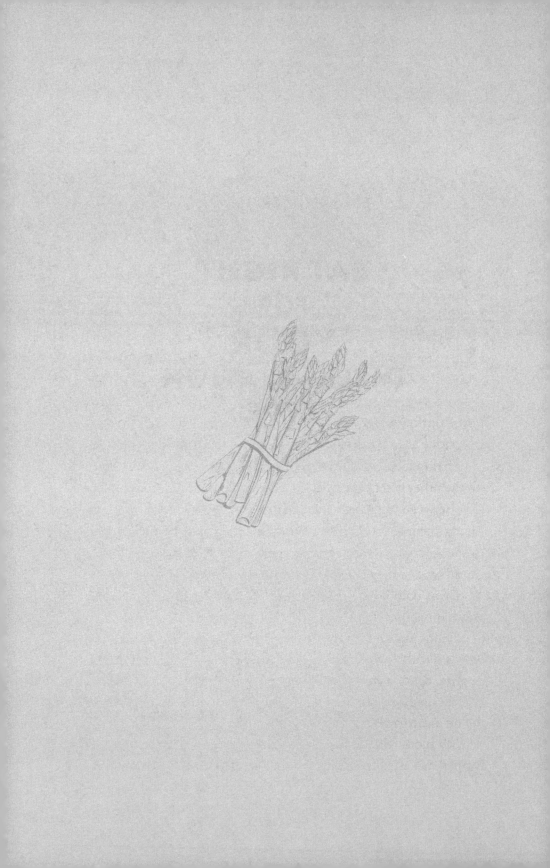

INTRODUCTION

I was packing for a trip to the lake. One minute, I was choosing clothes, folding them, and wedging them neatly into my duffel bag, feeling the excitement for a quick getaway with my boyfriend and his family, and thinking about what shade of coral to paint my nails. The next minute, I reached for my favorite swimsuit and a wave of dizziness came out of nowhere. I tried to steady myself, but the room started to spin. I began to black out, a darkness creeping in from my periphery as I fumbled for my phone to call my mom because my roommate wasn't home.

Shaking, I pressed the speed dial. "Hello? Maggie?" she asked on the other end of the line. I opened my mouth, but the connection between the words I wanted to say and my mouth actually saying them short-circuited. Nothing came out. I willed myself to speak, trying harder, trying to ask for help, and when I finally found words, they slurred together into complete gibberish.

I was completely shocked and scared. I didn't know what was happening.

I hung up and anxiously tried to text her instead, but the words hardly looked like words. I remember continuing to try. Typing, send. Typing, send. My phone's typing board blurred together, a haze of c's and d's, and the room continued to take me on a carousel of dizziness and confusion.

My mom called back. I answered but still no "real" words formed as I tried to speak. She told me bluntly: "Get to the ER, now." She didn't have a clue what was going on, and neither did I. Fortunately, my roommate got back just at that moment, and she rushed me to the ER. By the time I was in the ER bed, hooked to IVs and prepping for an MRI, MRA, and echo scan of my head and heart, the room had stabilized a bit. I was still dizzy and confused and my words weren't coming out quite right, but I felt better. Just as I was beginning to feel embarrassed, like I'd made a big deal out of nothing, the doctor came back in.

"Maggie, it looks like you had a TIA," he informed me calmly. A TIA, a transient ischemic attack, is a ministroke. Blood flow to your brain becomes either reduced or blocked, causing stroke-like symptoms such as garbled speech and severe dizziness.

I couldn't wrap my head around it. A ministroke? I was twenty-four, active, and had always been conscientious about making the healthiest choices. My friends turned to me for nutrition and health advice. How could this be?

The truth is, deep down I knew I had been severely "off" with my health for years. I was vibrant and healthy on the outside, but secretly struggling on the inside. Nearly three years prior, I had started to experience severe bloating. Even a snack like veggies with olive oil or hummus with gluten-free crackers would cause uncomfortable bloating in which my stomach would be hard to the touch. And one year prior, I'd faced a peak of my mental stress that had started to take a toll on my body. I was finishing the last three weeks of the first year of my nurse practitioner program at Vanderbilt University, when I had to move into a friend's house. The lease on my own place was up, and I had a few finals left to take before I'd head home, where I would complete my final year of the program as a "distance student"—which means I would be completing my final clinical experience in Indiana and going down once a month to Vanderbilt for what they call a "block week" for testing and on-site work.

In addition to the stress, my friend's house was nothing like what I was used to. I went from having one roommate to five roommates in a cramped space. They stayed up late into the night and had starkly different eating habits, including downing big tubs of Moose Tracks ice cream and greasy pizzas galore. I'm all for that here and there, but it was a combination of the food, the late nights, the stress, the pushing my mind and my body to the brink. I started to really struggle. I fell into their lifestyle because there was no room in the fridge for my food, and my usual 4:30 a.m. alarm to go work out before classes would have woken them. This quick pivot in lifestyle was a far cry from my lifelong health-conscious habits and early bedtimes. To make matters worse, I was more stressed than I'd ever been. I was distraught with the indecisiveness about whether I should stay in Nashville after graduation or move back to my hometown to be with my boyfriend. Oh, and finals. The stress caused yo-yo dieting, so I'd eat healthy throughout the week, keeping my carb intake low per the online guidelines I was following from some workout blog I saw, then I would binge on the weekends (not to mention all the end-of-year celebrations with alcohol and sweets).

My body was running on "E." My mind was whirling. I was stressed, and I felt like my whole world was spinning out of control. I just needed to hit the "pause" button, be alone for a few weeks, and just be still. Like I needed everyone to just go away and let me collect myself—but I couldn't. Have you ever felt like that?

One day, I walked out of a lecture and noticed that my legs felt tingly and tight. I pulled up my pant leg and my stomach dropped. One of my legs had become massively swollen from the knee down. I was horrified. This had never happened before. I was on birth control at the time and I knew that deep vein thrombosis is a possible complication of the pill, which can cause swelling of one leg. I thought that must be what was happening, and I went straight to the school health clinic to be scanned. The scan came back negative, and my doctor gave me two prescriptions: Lasix, a diuretic to reduce the fluid retention, and ibuprofen, an anti-inflammatory medication to counteract the swelling. He didn't tell me why it had happened, nor did he ask me anything about my lifestyle, stress, or nutrition habits. He just told me the scan was normal and that I should take the medications to help the swelling go away.

Well, the pills helped for a little while, but then the swelling continued and took over other extremities of my body. My face was visibly puffy. My ankle and foot bones became indistinguishable under the swelling, and I began to develop pitting edema, where indents in my skin would stay pressed in like small pits wherever I'd press on my swollen arms and legs. It was horrifying and embarrassing. Not only did I appear puffy and swollen, but I felt miserable. I explain how I felt each day like a hangover, except I hadn't had any alcohol.

Ultimately, after the stressful decision-making process, I decided to return to my hometown after graduating to begin my career and life there. My graduation day was marked by worry about the severe swelling underneath my robe, and I tried to mask it with baggy clothes for other festivities. I put on a smile and enjoyed some drinks and food with my family, even though I knew I'd wake up the next day in misery from a "food hangover." "Just push through, Maggie," I told myself. "They'll be gone in a few days, and I can recoup and get my swelling down then. Put on a smile and just get through."

A few days later I was on my drive home to Indiana from Tennessee, my left leg propped up, resting on my car seat against the door. It was a seven-hour road trip, and I drove the whole way. When I finally arrived in Indiana, I stepped out of the car and could hardly walk. My left leg had a two-inch-deep lengthwise indent across my thigh—right where it had been resting on the side of the door. My right leg was so swollen it looked like it belonged to an elephant. I was terrified to see how swollen they were. I stumbled uncomfortably inside and elevated them for the rest of the night, and it took hours and hours to reduce the inflammation even slightly.

Once I was settled back home, none of the feelings of being unsettled abated, and the stress continued to impact my health.

And that's what led me to the fateful night when I had a ministroke while packing for the lake.

LIFE POST MINISTROKE

After fully assessing my health and chronic symptoms post-TIA, the doctors discharged me with a strong recommendation to follow up soon with my doctor or a cardiologist. I was told I'd need to see a specialist who could determine the root cause of what I was experiencing, since it hadn't yet been determined.

I wish I could say that I immediately found a specialist who helped me get to the bottom of everything. I wish that the TIA was the biggest of my worries, but it truly wasn't. My journey was far from over. The swelling, weight gain, fatigue, bloating, and overall sickness had taken over my entire life. I remember one trip during this time to Chicago for my boyfriend's birthday. I let myself take a break from the diet I had started to try to reduce the swelling and weight gain for that dinner, and simply ate what everyone else was having. I didn't want to seem "annoying" or picky, so I just went with the flow. The next morning I woke up, felt horrible, stumbled to the bathroom, and stepped on a scale, only to see a devastating and scary twelve-pound weight gain—literally overnight. I deleted those photos from my phone in an attempt to delete those memories—my face swollen tremendously, my body in physical pain like a bruise head to toe, and my brain fogged to the max.

I had hives all over my body that burned and itched. My heart raced, and tears rolled down my face when I'd catch myself in a mirror somewhere to see my body broken out, almost unrecognizable. My hair was thinning dramatically. I was freezing all the time. My bloating was painful and had me looking pregnant most every day. My natural, high-energy personality was dulled by a thick brain fog that rendered me constantly exhausted and distant. I continued to go through the ups and downs of dramatic overnight weight gain followed by days and days of trying to get it off again. Eventually the weight gain stayed, and my set point just kept getting higher and higher with each passing day. I felt like there was no hope and I'd never return to my normal self. I felt like my body was spinning out of control and I was screaming inside, but there was nothing I could do about it.

I'd have dizzy spells driving, where I would need to quickly pull my car over because my vision had started to blur and I thought I might pass out. Many times I ended up on the side of some road with tears in my eyes, scared to push that pedal to get back on the road and to wherever I was headed. I just wanted to be at home. I just wanted to soak in an Epsom salt bath, get in my baggy clothes, squeeze on some compression socks, prop my legs up on a big pile of pillows, pour peppermint oil on my rock-hard swollen belly, and lie in bed with no one to see me for days—my safe place.

The cycle continued.

I remember all those moments so vividly and yet they felt as if they were all just part of a scary dream. Even now, it's hard to imagine that this really happened to me.

My health decline impacted even what should have been my biggest and happiest moments, such as the day my now-husband proposed to me in October of 2015. The happy memories from the day I got engaged to the love of my life are clouded by the food restrictions, feeling sick, and looking swollen in all our photos. The photos from that day, from our engagement photo shoot, my bachelorette party, and even the wedding are tainted with those memories of uncertainty and fear. I don't even look like myself. My face was so swollen, causing my eyes to squint and my smile to shorten, and my clothes held tightly to my bloated body despite purchasing larger sizes to make up for my swelling. By that time, I had gained nearly forty pounds in about one year from all the imbalances and inflammation.

I went to so many doctors' appointments, I lost count. They bounced me around like a basketball. I was just another number on their list of patients to get through that day, only to send me along to the next person.

I went to my first cardiologist appointment hopeful. Nothing came of it. They thought it was my hormones, so I was referred to an endocrinologist.

I went to the endocrinologist appointment hopeful. Nothing came of it. They referred me to an immunologist and allergist.

And the process continued.

I showed up hopeful to every appointment I had, believing that this time would be different. This time I would finally know *something*. I would even hope that they'd find cancer. At least then we would finally know what it was.

It all ended when I met my immunologist and allergist. He was good—I liked him. He drew a handful of blood vials on my first visit, and he told me he'd try to get to the bottom of this. When I returned for my follow-up, he looked at the labs, looked at me, then looked at the labs again. "Maggie," he said slowly, "it looks like you have a rare kidney disease . . ."

I was frightened by the words but relieved by the diagnosis. Finally, someone had determined what was going on. And if there was a diagnosis, there could be a corresponding treatment plan. There was a way through.

But then he continued.

"Truthfully, I'm one of the best specialists in my field, and I really don't know why this is happening. There's no explanation. I wish I could tell you more, but I simply don't know why your kidneys are failing," he leveled with me. "You also have a severe immunodeficiency disorder, and your protein levels are also extremely low. I expect that you'll be on IV immunoglobulin for the rest of your life."

I understood the gravity of what he was telling me, but at least we had more clarity (or so I thought). After being referred from specialist to specialist, I felt like I finally had found a physician who could help. He turned to the nurse to explain the next steps.

"Schedule a follow-up appointment for Maggie for six months from now to check in on things," he told her, then shook my hand and walked back to his office.

Six months?! He offered ZERO advice on what to do in those six months. Zero discussion about my horrible symptoms that left me feeling like a zombie sleepwalking through life. Zero answers. I scheduled my appointment looking down, holding back my frustration. I rushed out of the office to the parking lot, breathing slowly to try to stall the cascade of tears until I could settle into the privacy and comfort of my car. And once I sat down in the driver's seat and closed the door, I began to sob.

I sobbed for the six months of blank space ahead of me until I could see the specialist again. I sobbed for the diagnoses he had given me, without any real treatment plan or help on what to do next. I sobbed because I had thought he would be my answer at last and truly help me get to the bottom of it. I sobbed for every specialist I'd believed in who couldn't tell me what was wrong.

I sobbed for the ambiguity of my health, which was leaving my life in total disarray. I sobbed for the chaos that my body was going through. I sobbed for how alone and hopeless I felt—if no one, not even one of the top medical specialists in the *world*, could properly identify what was going on, when would it end?

I took a deep breath and pulled myself together. "Enough is enough," I decided with conviction. I was done. I was tired of putting hope in doctors who couldn't tell me what was wrong. No one was going to care about me or my health as much as I do. I was in charge now, and I was taking back control.

That moment of "enough is enough" pivoted the course of my life forever. With my mom's encouragement, I enrolled at the Institute for Functional Medicine's full Functional Medicine Certification program for licensed healthcare providers. Since I was already a nurse practitioner, I was able to apply to its program and was thrilled to find I was accepted and would begin school yet again—which wasn't on my "agenda" after just recently graduating from Vanderbilt with my master's, but I was determined to get to the bottom of what was going on in my body, since conventional medicine had failed me tremendously.

I knew I liked the functional/integrative model of healing the body. I did see some functional and integrative practitioners in my bounce to different specialists, but these particular practitioners weren't treating my individual imbalances, and were instead giving out one-size-fits-all diet and supplement plans. It was just like conventional medicine, handing me a pill for my symptoms and abnormal values. You should have seen my cabinet of endless supplements!

I did still believe in the functional and integrative model, though, because of my mom. She had been diagnosed with stage 3 colon cancer when she was just thirty-six years old. Her doctors had told her they couldn't do anything more for her. She asked God for a sign, to see if she should keep fighting for her life. He delivered. She knew that God was telling her it was not her time to go.

So she made a vow to heal herself, much as I did that afternoon in the immunologist's parking lot. She went away for some time to get treatment at the Cancer Treatment Centers of America, which had an integrative approach to health and used a combination of aromatherapy, touch, nutritional eating, and holistic medicine (in addition to chemotherapy) to beat cancer. Decades later, my mom is still cancer-free.

Now, it's important to understand that I am not against conventional medicine. We need conventional medicine. I am so grateful for the doctor who saved my first child's life by deciding to give me an emergency C-section. I am so grateful for the nurses who revived him when he was born with no signs of life: no heartbeat, no breathing, no response to stimulation, no muscle tone, and covered in purple. I'm grateful we have antibiotics when a bacterial infection rages in our bodies. For surgeons who save people every day during a heart attack, after a gun wound, or after a car accident. For the pharmaceuticals we have that help people relieve their excruciating pain, treat their debilitating depression, or calm their unbearable bowels to bridge the gap between healing their body and just getting through the day. But the fact is that conventional medicine, although needed in some situations, does a great disservice to those with chronic aches, pains, and nagging symptoms. It does a disservice to most of the chronic diseases in the world today, and the inflammatory conditions explored in this book. In conventional medicine, the real answers aren't being discovered to uncover root causes of disease. The doctors and practitioners aren't allotted enough time to spend with their patients to reconnect with them and help them day-to-day. The support isn't there for accessibility and lasting change. Insurance companies help with medications, but not with the lifestyle things that can really help a person thrive and achieve wellness.

A GUIDE TO FUNCTIONAL MEDICINE

The Institute for Functional Medicine opened my eyes to holistic health and well-being in a way that changed me. I dove in and got to work, attending conferences, listening to lectures, researching, reading, and studying. As it turns out, there was a root to every diagnosis I'd been given and every symptom I'd experienced. I didn't "have" all those diagnoses my doctors had plagued me with.

What I had was *inflammation*. Inflammation that was causing a decline and imbalance in almost all the systems of my body as a *whole*. The body is not segmented; all of its systems are connected. And I started to learn to ask "WHY." Why did I have inflammation? What was the root cause of it for my unique story? Not a single medication or supplement that I'd been prescribed during my health journey up to this point was treating the root cause of the inflammation, just all the many, many symptoms I had: bloating, constipation, fatigue, headaches, skin breakouts, swelling, weight gain, and dizziness. True healing

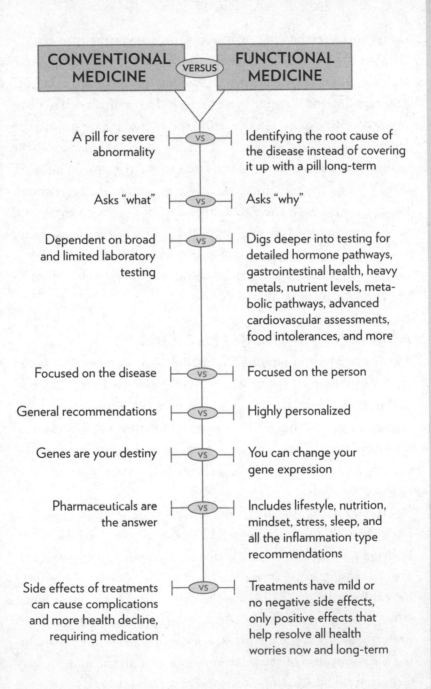

CONVENTIONAL MEDICINE — VERSUS — FUNCTIONAL MEDICINE

CONVENTIONAL MEDICINE	VS	FUNCTIONAL MEDICINE
A pill for severe abnormality	VS	Identifying the root cause of the disease instead of covering it up with a pill long-term
Asks "what"	VS	Asks "why"
Dependent on broad and limited laboratory testing	VS	Digs deeper into testing for detailed hormone pathways, gastrointestinal health, heavy metals, nutrient levels, metabolic pathways, advanced cardiovascular assessments, food intolerances, and more
Focused on the disease	VS	Focused on the person
General recommendations	VS	Highly personalized
Genes are your destiny	VS	You can change your gene expression
Pharmaceuticals are the answer	VS	Includes lifestyle, nutrition, mindset, stress, sleep, and all the inflammation type recommendations
Side effects of treatments can cause complications and more health decline, requiring medication	VS	Treatments have mild or no negative side effects, only positive effects that help resolve all health worries now and long-term

begins by identifying the root of inflammation for your specific body and story.

I finally had the answers I was looking for. I wiped my white-board clean (figuratively), and I started fresh with a set plan to target and combat the causes of my inflammation.

It worked.

Today I no longer suffer from a "mystery disease" or experience any of the devastating symptoms that had rendered me so helpless. I'm not on any medications anymore, either. I no longer swell up after eating certain foods. I maintain a balanced and healthy diet with ease, and I don't feel restricted in any way. Both my energy and my personality are back and better than ever, and despite being told by top specialists that I was infertile, I'm the proud mother of three beautiful children.

Once I learned to target the root causes of my own inflammation, I knew I had a responsibility to help others in the same way I'd helped myself. So I left my hospital job in conventional medicine and started my own online health consulting business to work one-on-one with clients from all around the world and help them regain control of their health. My clients often come to me feeling the same way I felt all those years ago: frustrated, confused, wrestling with "mystery symptoms," and sick of being told "everything is normal" or to take a pill for their symptoms. They've usually tried everything, or so it seems, and nothing works long-term to get them the results they're after.

Through targeting inflammation, clients have resolved chronic insomnia and pain, reversed autoimmune disorders, healed gut imbalances, shrunk tumor sizes, overcome anxiety and depression, canceled surgeries that were no longer needed, become pregnant despite being told they were infertile, lost weight effortlessly, and regained control from the nagging symptoms that originally stole their day-to-day health, presence, and happiness.

That's why this book is all about targeting your unique root cause of inflammation—your inflammation type! Based on what I've learned, discovered, and applied, I knew I had to create an accessible guide for all people—regardless of age, race, lifestyle, or current health status—who are struggling with chronic illness and undiagnosable symptoms and want to regain their sense of control. I can't work one-on-one with everyone, but I can share my knowledge and expertise with each and every single one of you, and that's exactly why I knew I had an obligation and responsibility to YOU to write this book. You deserve these answers and guidance, and although we are not face-to-face right now, please know that I am thinking of you holding this book, reading these words, and truly changing your life for the better from this moment forward. I am SO proud of you, and excited to see what all this opens up for you in your life. This book is a solution-oriented guide to help you transform your lifestyle, reduce inflammation, and get back to who you are with more energy and vibrancy than ever. It's the guide I wish I could have given my twenty-four-year-old self.

By the end of this book, you'll understand what exactly inflammation is, what it does, and what happens when it becomes chronic. We will target your inflammation in a series of solution-oriented chapters, helping you better understand how your environment, diet, habits, mental health, and lifestyle can contribute to the inflammation you're experiencing. This is a book intended to help you reflect on everything that may be causing inflammation, so that you will be equipped with the necessary tools to step into vibrant health! From this place of understanding, you'll be able to change your choices and lifestyle and experience a complete transformation of your health, productivity, and energy.

And possibly of most importance, through the recommendations and knowledge you will gain in the pages of this book, you will boost your immune system and actually rewire your body to be stronger than ever before. You will build a strong and mighty immune system that will help to protect you against anything that comes your way in the future—whether it be a virus, bacteria, excess stress, toxicity, trauma, or even a pregnancy. Your body's immune system will be supercharged to help you thrive through it all!

The symptoms you've been experiencing have lasted too long. You deserve to stand in your full power without the discomfort and pain. The world deserves you at your best—in complete, unwavering, and exalting wellness. The ripple effect when you yourself are fully well will impact every being who may cross your path. You will positively impact your coworkers, your family, your unborn children, and the world in full. I'm here for you and rooting for you!

So, what do you say? Let's blast that inflammation for good!

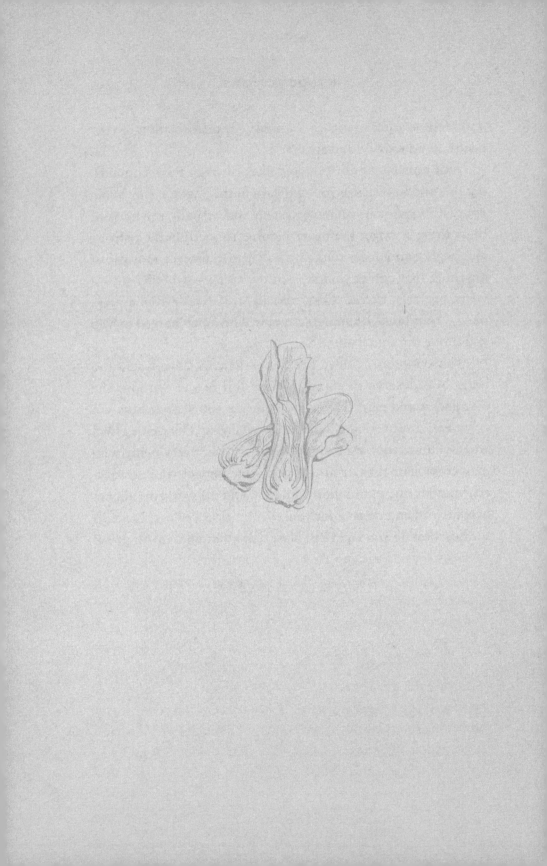

1

UNDERSTANDING HOW INFLAMMATION WORKS IN YOUR BODY

et's start with the million-dollar question: What exactly *is* inflammation? Well, I'll begin by setting a record straight: inflammation itself is not the enemy. Sure, this book is all about curing inflammation, but it goes deeper than that. Rather, it's the root causes of inflammation, and the long-term impact chronic inflammation can have on the body, that can act as secret killers.

To understand inflammation, think back to a time you were stung by a bee. Ouch! Aside from the initial sting from the bee, you likely remember that the area became red and swollen, and was burning and throbbing, with a soreness and continued swelling.

Those symptoms were part of an acute inflammatory response, which is considered a "healthy physiological response aimed at wound healing."[1] Your body leaps into action to fight against the foreign substance that's threatening your body from the cut, abrasion, sting, or other wound that you endure. What causes the redness and swelling isn't the bee's stinger itself, but your body's defensive response to the sting and injury. Inflammation is your body's response to an offender in its attempt to survive.

Your body also kicks off an immediate inflammatory response when you get acutely sick. When you have a virus, a foreign pathogen attacks your body, and your body goes into full defense mode to protect you. One of the ways it does this is by invoking a fever to kill the virus (which is another type of inflammation). We need this. We need a strong immune system and inflammatory response to help us in these situations, for sure.

The problem is that our bodies are not inflamed just to acute situations like a beesting, but are in "inflammatory mode" and thus damaging our immune systems almost all day every day, year after year, due to various offending stressors that are placed on our bodies in today's modern world. This is what causes chronic illness and the nagging horrible symptoms you may have.

THE CAUSES OF INFLAMMATION

The causes of inflammation can include both infectious and noninfectious factors. The following table from the journal *Oncotarget* lists the etiologies of inflammation.[2]

Infectious factors (those that make us sick) include:

■ Bacteria
■ Viruses
■ Microorganisms

Noninfectious factors could be:

■ Physical (physical injury, burns, frostbite, trauma, radiation, and foreign bodies [including that beesting])

- Chemical (glucose, fatty acids, toxins, alcohol, chemical irritants)
- Biological (damaged cells)
- Psychological (excitement or stress)

Inflammation is simply your body's way of fighting against these injurious stimuli. When one of these factors enters or nears the body and poses a threat, a chemical response activates the release of leukocyte chemotaxis, which produce inflammatory *cytokines*.

Cytokines are secreted by the cells of your immune system to regulate immunity and inflammation. In nonmedical jargon, your body releases chemical soldiers to fight against the bad guys (pathogens and toxins), and the weapon those soldiers use to fight them is *inflammation*. Although the weapon is useful in attacking those toxins and bad guys, it also ruins the battlefield and some of the good guys. The body and the immune system take a hit when inflammation goes off, and both are greatly damaged when this process is happening each day.

The stressors, and the "bad guys," are impossible to avoid completely, so if you aren't decreasing your overall inflammation, and also working to boost your immune system every single day, your "battlefield" will become toxic, barren, and deadly. Your body will crash, and instead of feeling and looking vibrant and energetic, you'll be like the dark and barren field without the resources to regain yourself.

HOW DOES INFLAMMATION HELP US?

Like I stated above, we *need* inflammation. Inflammation has an essential purpose to keep us safe and sometimes can even save our lives. When these acute inflammatory responses occur, it's simply the body doing its job.

There are five cardinal signs of inflammation: redness, swelling, heat, pain, and loss of function.[3] Each of these is a by-product of your body's attempts to heal or protect you when infection or injury occurs.

Then, cytokines and other inflammation-inducing chemicals dilate blood vessels so that your plasma and immune cells can more swiftly get to the site of the injury or infection. Think of this as widening the tunnels on a highway so more "cars" (or, in this case, immune cells and plasma) can get through more quickly. "The sensation of heat is caused by the increased movement of blood through dilated vessels," which also contributes to redness.

Swelling occurs as a "result of the increased passage of fluid into surrounding tissues," as well as the infiltration of the cells to the damaged area. When plasma and defensive cells rush to the affected area, they cause swelling simply because of the increased amount of fluid.

Once at the site, the major cells of the immune system get to work. Antibodies and platelets stop the bleeding if there's been a cut to the skin, and also attack any microorganisms. Then, neutrophils, which are a type of phagocyte (a white blood cell that surrounds and absorbs bacteria), get to work removing any further threats. A whole team works within your body to take care of you and protect you.

Pain can happen as a result of the initial damage (such as in the case of a beesting) or "the stretching of sensory nerves due to oedema." Oedema (or edema) refers to the excess of fluids in the tissues of the body—again, all fluids that are helping to heal you. The edema or the pain can also contribute to the loss of function, as can the replacement of functional cells with scar tissue.

Edema can also look like visual swelling in the body. For example, when I first was struggling with my own health complications in my early twenties, edema was one of my major symptoms that was most noticeable. I'd swell up "like a balloon," I'd always say. Truly. My legs, arms, and face would have so much excess fluid in them that I appeared massively swollen, and if you pressed on my skin it would leave a huge indent, known as pitting edema, from all the fluid. It was horrifying and so terrible to deal with. But note that my body, and likely yours, was not inflaming in this way due to a beesting and then going back to "normal"; it was a chronic and long-lasting response due to the excess stressors I was dealing with. My body was in inflammation overdrive.

While it's important and helpful when part of an acute response, it's worth noting that inflammation acts in a way that should be short-term oriented and actually helpful for our defense mechanisms. However, the more your body engages in an inflammatory response, the more damaging it can be in the long run. Dr. David Agus from the University of Southern California's Department of Medicine noted that every time you get a fever—a normal, acute inflammatory response to a virus—it increases your chances of having cancer or heart disease down the road.[4] Yikes! And this also decreases our immune system function due to the added stress and toll it takes on our body. Our bodies are programmed to care about survival *right now*, and when danger strikes in the form of a pathogen or toxic compound, your immune system immediately goes into attack mode to protect you, even though inflammation can hurt your health down the line. This is a horrible and messy cycle that we MUST put an end to or your world, our world, will never truly heal.

Reducing inflammation and spreading positivity are two of the most important things you can do each day.

WHEN INFLAMMATION BECOMES CHRONIC

The real danger of inflammation is when it becomes *chronic*. When day after day we are setting off our internal inflammatory responses not just to a beesting but to nearly everything—a fight with your spouse; anger in traffic; fear and worry; toxins in our food, air, water, hygiene, and household products; poor eating habits; lack of sleep; and a sedentary lifestyle. This all leads to chronic inflammation, and all the many nagging symptoms and diseases you now experience. Anxiety, depression, pain, insomnia, bloating, diarrhea/constipation, skin breakouts, hair thinning, migraines and headaches, even cancers, organ dysfunction, autoimmunity, and diseases, all can be linked back to chronic inflammation and the corresponding impacts it has within our body.

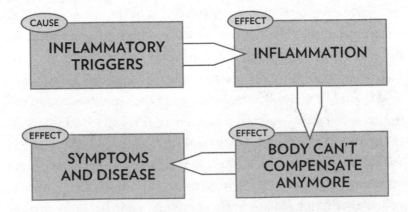

According to the journal article "Obesity and Inflammation: The Linking Mechanism and the Complications," chronic inflammation differs from acute inflammation in that "it lasts for a long time and is characterized by the presence of lymphocytes and macrophages and the proliferation of blood vessels and connective tissue."[5] OK, now let's translate that into plain ole English, shall we? This essentially just means that inflammation that should be short-term continues for a really long time, which causes a whole bunch of problems in our health long-term. It also builds up, so the more inflammatory triggers you have, the more total inflammation is within your body, the less your body can compensate, and the more symptoms and diseases will develop.

When chronic, inflammation shifts from a healthy, normal response that is confined to the acute response time of responding to a wound or a sickness to a constant defense response. In a chronically inflammatory state, the body continues to attack *anything* it deems as toxic, and since you are presented with so many toxins in our day-to-day world—we all are—it wages a constant war within your body. You may not even know it is happening until your symptoms start to show up in bigger ways. You may even feel "healthy" and "fine" right now, but inside your body is telling a completely different story, and it's only a matter of time until you crash if it's not resolved.

This chronic inflammation can be from things like allergens and toxins in your environment, your mental state, food, and toxic ingredients in your household and hygiene items such as soap, lotion, cleaners, and makeup.

While redness, swelling, heat, pain, and loss of function seem similar to what we'd see externally after a beesting or in other cases of an abrasion or injury to the skin, chronic instances of inflammation more than likely happen internally and can contribute to autoimmune diseases, poor gastrointestinal function, food intolerances, headaches, anxiety, depression, sleep and energy complications, among other nagging symptoms and diseases. In other words, all the things that make you feel unwell . . . or like you want to press the snooze button another five times because you just can't gather the energy, motivation, and drive to get up and get through another day of aches, pains, and frustrating symptoms. This is no way to live. You deserve better, and I believe you can reach that new level of vibrant health—it's here for you!

Conditions that result from chronic inflammation can include:

- Irritable bowel syndrome, inflammatory bowel disease, diarrhea/constipation, gut pain
- Rheumatoid arthritis, osteoarthritis
- Psoriasis, eczema, acne
- Multiple sclerosis
- Atherosclerosis

As well as:

- Hormonal imbalances—PMS, lack of periods, heavy periods, irregular periods, low thyroid, infertility, adrenal insufficiency
- Anxiety, depression, worry
- Headaches and migraines
- Insomnia, fatigue

Some of the above are considered in conventional medicine to be "inflammatory disorders."[6] Beyond these disorders, *Chronic Inflammation* notes that "chronic inflammation has been directly implicated in a wide range of degenerative human health disorders. These pathologies encompass almost all of present-day noncommunicable diseases such as obesity, diabetes, atherosclerosis, and high blood pressure, as well as cancer."[7]

Additionally, autoimmune diseases such as Hashimoto's thyroiditis occur when inflammation mistakenly targets and kills the body's own *healthy* cells and tissue, believing that they are pathogens.

So, although inflammation is a good thing when it's part of an acute response, the chronic presence of inflammation is turning out to be a major cause of almost every chronic disease and nagging symptom! It's also at the root of what I call "mystery illnesses," when a host of unidentifiable and odd symptoms are experienced with no explained diagnosis as to why. Not to mention how we respond to things like viruses.

An inflamed body and weakened immune system simply cannot handle all of the toxicity, viruses, mental stress, and poor lifestyle choices we're exposed to today, and eventually it will stop being able to compensate and will crash. We must strengthen the internal environment of our body in order to get well and stay well.

The more inflammation that occurs *now*, the higher the chances are that you will develop heart disease, cancer, or other complications down the road. If one fever can increase your chances, imagine how heightened your chances are when you're dealing with chronic inflammation! When heart disease, cancer, or other noncommunicable diseases arise, they are likely due to chronic inflammation that has been occurring internally for a long time. This is also the case with premature aging—no thank you! By addressing inflammation, we can "age backward," not just in regard to the vibrant state of our skin but also in our brain health, heart health, and internal functions. By addressing inflammation, we give our body the tools to thrive year after year.

YOUR "TOTAL TOXIC BURDEN"

When I was constantly swelling, fatigued, gaining weight, stressed out, feeling down, and bloated—BLAH—it was the result of my own chronic inflammation. I say it happened "all of a sudden," but really the accumulation of years' worth of toxicities and stressors led my body to that state of health decline. A number of contributing factors had been causing damage beneath the surface for a long time, and the major symptoms just didn't show up until my body was at its absolute breaking point. I now refer to your body's ability to handle these toxic offenders as your "Total Toxic Burden," which is a phrase I learned at the Institute for Functional Medicine and throughout many of my studies that really stuck with me. It helped me understand this mechanism of taxing my body. Your body can compensate for being under "attack" by outside stressors for a long time, but eventually, the body cannot compensate any longer, and those small symptoms you'd been ignoring, which have been slowly creeping in, exaggerate big-time. Essentially, you've hit your "max," and your body says, "NOPE! Not today, Maggie—we're done."

Once I learned about all the things in our life that can cause chronic inflammation, toxicity, and a crash in our immune system, all I could think was, "No wonder I'm sick!" Honestly, I'm surprised that my "crash" in my early twenties didn't happen sooner. My poor body was working in overdrive for far too long. But no one told me. No one warned me. No one talks about this stuff—it's not "sexy" or "cool" to talk about how certain chemicals, the air quality, food, and even your own mindset can chemically imbalance and harm your body. Especially when you're a twenty-one-year-old in college. I could not believe the choices I had been making, now that I know what our diet, stress, and environment can do to our body. I was pushing my body to the max, and the poor thing just couldn't compensate any longer. I'm sorry, body! Thank you, thank you for taking care of me for so long even when I wasn't treating you the best.

At the onset of my symptoms, I was under an incredible amount of mental stress from the indecision I was facing regarding my postgrad plans. When stressed, your body goes into a fight-or-flight response, which naturally causes inflammation even when you don't need it physically. The fight-or-flight response sends your body into survival mode and kicks off the same internal response that would happen if you encountered a bear on a hike—it freaks out and does whatever it can to save you. Your body can't tell the difference between one type of threat and another. It just knows that it's stressed, and it reacts accordingly. We'll talk more about how mental stress causes inflammation in chapter 6.

Back when I was in school, I was putting my body under additional pressure even beyond school itself. I would wake up super early (4:30–5:00 a.m.) to get in an intense workout before classes. I was then rushing home after the workout, rushing to get ready, rushing off to school, sitting down and using a lot of brain power all day long, working through lunch, then sometimes even going to another workout at night (hot yoga was my evening workout of choice), then studying until I basically couldn't keep my eyes open any longer and fell asleep. That was my day. Beyond that, I'd jam-pack my weekends with to-dos or trips with friends, one too many cocktails and pieces of pizza, and still be in a sympathetic state of "always on the go." I rarely would allow my brain and body to just rest. Even when I took time to go "relax" in the sauna, it wasn't really to unwind; I wanted to multitask and get a sweat or soak in while I answered texts and emails and got some work done. I was also yo-yo dieting: bouncing between bingeing on unhealthy foods on the weekend and eating strict through the week, usually following online workout diets that eliminated most carbohydrates and fats and included the same foods day in and out—broccoli, skinless boneless chicken breast, and tilapia, anyone? Although externally I looked healthy, vibrant, and fit, I was running my body ragged, which was sending its inflammatory response haywire and weakening my immune system. I was playing with a ticking time bomb, and it was only a matter of time until it would explode.

Nutrition was a really big part of my story and health decline. Every time I ate processed or high-sugar foods, each bite of a white flour–laden cupcake or a greasy slice of pizza was yet another "offender" adding up to my own Total Toxic Burden. The toxicity goes beyond traditional inflammatory food (such as fried, processed, or high-sugar foods), as there can be toxins in foods we believe are healthy. Even a bite of an apple can have toxins in it that will cause an inflammatory response if it was sprayed with harmful chemicals and not washed thoroughly before consuming. I don't say this to scare you, but to show that there is so much more at play than you may realize. Even if you think you eat "healthy" according to the typical prescription of what healthy food looks like, toxins can still sneak in. And further, even if there aren't toxins in that apple (because you chose an organic apple and washed it thoroughly), in today's world it unfortunately may not have the level of nutrients in it that an apple should have due to the lack of nutrients in the soil in which it was grown. AND—even if it had no toxins, and had many nutrients—if your own body doesn't digest it well (maldigestion) or absorb it well (malabsorption), you'll still be missing out on what should be wonderful fruit to boost your immune system and lead to health.

The inflammation I was experiencing came from smaller things I didn't ever think about, too—things beyond food and mental stress, such as the heavily scented lotion I wore every day that had inflammatory chemicals in it, the water I'd drink (despite using a popular refrigerator filter, which unbeknownst to me at the time didn't filter my water properly), and even the air in my apartment because I didn't have an air filter regulating toxins in the air. The compilation of all these offenders topped my Total Toxic Burden, leading to my steep health decline.

THE ROLE OF GENETICS

You may wonder why someone like your spouse or best friend can eat all the same things you do, live in the same apartment, drink the same water from the tap, use the same products, and *not* show the same symptoms that you have. Or, how some people can get extremely sick and even die from a virus, while others seem to easily recover after a few days of rest. This is where genetics combined with lifestyle choices can play a role in determining how inflammation shows up in your body. Your genetics can predispose you to certain health concerns down the road. It may make it harder for your body to do something— like metabolize coffee, use vitamin B, or stabilize sugars— than another person's body. That said, genetics alone do not mean you *will* or *will not* "have" or "get" a certain disease or health complication. It's the lifestyle factors and inflammatory offenders that may activate and turn on the risk factors you may already be genetically predisposed to have.

In addition, our body may have certain systems and/or organs that are more susceptible to decline. Not to sound too harsh toward ourselves, but it could be that there are certain areas in our body that are "weaker" than others. These areas are the ones that typically express imbalances when things go awry. For me, my weakest areas are my thyroid and my hormones—hands down. Both my mom and my grandma had struggles with low thyroid, and I had always had hormonal dysregulation. In fact, I didn't have my first menstrual cycle until it was medically induced with birth control pills at age eighteen! Yup. Looking back, I can see clearly that my body had been out of balance long before I knew it. My mom definitely had a hunch that something was "off" with me back then, but no doctors would listen to her. She took me to multiple doctors' appointments to test my thyroid and hormones and I had so many scans of my uterus and abdomen, but everything always looked "normal" on tests, so we just didn't do anything about it. Not only did I not have periods, but I was always freezing cold. You'd find me in fuzzy socks, sweats, and a sweatshirt with the hood strings pulled so tight around my face you could just see a peep of my eyes and nose. I'd be wrapped tight like a burrito in the heaviest blankets we had, all while my other siblings were chilling in their shorts and T-shirts. I personally remember that I was always hungry. I could never get full, it seemed! Clearly there was something going on inside me even before I had any "real" symptoms that worried me enough. Over time, the hormonal imbalances kept getting worse and worse despite me having no idea of what was going on inside my body. I didn't know that every time I was stressed out, didn't sleep well, or ate a bunch of junk, I was putting fuel on the fire that would eventually spread far and wide. So, when my Total Toxic Burden met its max capacity and my body could no longer compensate, the inflammatory storm showed up through thyroid and hormonal issues first. The thing is, though, the body is all connected. No organ or body part is disconnected from another. When there are imbalances in one area, all the other areas are negatively affected as well. That explains why when you're struggling with the symptoms you're struggling with, it's absolutely essential to address the body and healing through a holistic and whole-body lens, rather than addressing just that one specific organ. It's also why when conventional medicine gives you a pharmaceutical medication to help with your symptoms, it's rarely ever the answer. Let's take my case as an example. My thyroid was "off," yes. My cycles were irregular. Conventional medicine would tell me, "Here, take this thyroid medicine for your thyroid, and birth control to help your periods." Done. This model didn't look further to ask WHY my body was having imbalance in these areas and then HOW to fix it. This model didn't consider all the other body systems that were impacted by these things, such as my levels of nutrients or amino acids, my metabolism, gut health status, or detoxification pathways. This is where a huge hole lies in conventional medicine. Again, very useful for some things, but absolutely lacking where many of us need it most.

In the next chapter, you'll take an assessment to determine your inflammation type. Again, I want to be clear that I do not believe genetics are the "cause" of your inflammation or health concerns, but rather they may predispose you to being more likely to develop certain symptoms, diseases, or imbalances if your Total Toxic Burden and inflammatory stressors hit their maximum capacity and your internal environment falls under attack.

HOW TO GET RID OF INFLAMMATION

I know that all of this information can be quite overwhelming, so I'll skip to the good news: *inflammation is under your control*. You are not at the whim of some outside influences that will render you unwell and frustrated forever! We get to choose how we breathe, move, think, and live. We get to choose what we do to either hurt or heal our internal environment in order to combat inflammation, reduce toxic exposure, and allow our body to heal itself. In fact, that's what the main goal is—for us to give our body a helping hand in the right direction by reducing the inflammation and toxicities we put on our body, so it can do its job and heal itself. Our body is far smarter than any doctor or pill in the world. Once we know the factors that contribute to our inflammation, we can make strategic changes in our lifestyle that will allow us to return to the vibrant state of health we so deserve! Everyone has a different Total Toxic Burden, and everyone can either eliminate or add to their burden with the smaller choices they make. Picking up this book was a powerful first step toward changing your external and internal environments to reduce inflammation for good! Take time right this second to acknowledge that. You, my friend, have just taken the step that may very well change your life for the better forever. I'm so proud of you!

The conventional model of medicine will prescribe medications or one-size-fits-all diets, and even perform surgeries to mask the symptoms of inflammation rather than address the root cause. The problem with this is that they are just Band-Aids that attempt to cover up the symptoms or make some lab value appear "better," and they don't actually address the deeper issues. A metaphor I like to use to explain this is that inflammation is like a leak in your fridge. Imagine that the leak has been slowly ruining the beautiful hardwood floors in your kitchen. The floors are looking rough, so you replace them. But then, after more time goes by, your new floors are ruined just like before because the leak—or the root cause—wasn't fixed! You never addressed WHY the floors were ruined, and so the damage is just being covered up and will happen again and again.

Now let's get more concrete with an example in the body. If you have low thyroid levels, you can take a thyroid pill to raise them. But if the cause of the low thyroid isn't addressed, the actual problem is still happening, and although your labs may look improved, the inflammation in your body is still going haywire and causing long-term damage in ALL your systems and organs. You're never actually fixing the symptoms or abnormalities, you're covering them up, which leads to much greater problems down the road.

Same with bloating, constipation, diarrhea. Your doctor will likely give you a pill to help combat these symptoms, but will never address why they're happening in the first place in order to fix the core problem so you don't have to deal with these sometimes debilitating, embarrassing, painful, and frustrating symptoms. It just doesn't make sense.

Here's the question I want you to get used to asking yourself: What caused the inflammation that you're experiencing in the first place? Then what caused that? And what caused that? This is the mindset to use when addressing your health, rather than focusing on symptoms and abnormalities alone. I want to be clear that the "leak" or the "inflammation" still isn't the root of these symptoms, but it's a part of the story. The "leak" didn't just magically appear one day. Something had been going on causing damage slowly behind the scenes for a while—your body's reaction to something, whether it's the fragrance of your favorite perfume, the heavy smog outside your city apartment, or a food intolerance you didn't know about. We must find out now what that "something" or series of somethings is for you. What stressor caused the inflammation? And, usually, it's not just one single thing, it's a combination of stressors that adds up and eventually becomes too much for your body to handle any further, which causes the ultimate destruction and corresponding symptoms or disease.

With my three-step plan to address inflammation and the root causes of your nagging symptoms and health complications, not only will we address what you eat, but we will take a unique look at your environment, the products you use, how you breathe, your mindset, your sleep habits, and even the water you drink. Most of all, we will keep this SIMPLE. Listen—I'm here for you. You've been through a lot already. You've bawled your eyes out, you've felt hopeless, you've been let down, you've been in pain. You've been on this roller coaster for far too long, and I'm here to hold your hand and help you through this—to help you finally feel the way you deserve to feel—FREE.

This book isn't going to be a strict rule book with restrictions for what you can or can't do—I'm not for that. I want you to absolutely thrive in this modern world, and enjoy every moment of life to the fullest, in a way that will keep your internal body and mind at their optimal performance. This is a guide that will *empower* you to understand every factor that can lead to your Total Toxic Burden, so you're able to make choices in alignment with what matters most to you and live your life to the absolute fullest.

You get to choose what to focus on in your life in order to feel, look, and perform your very best. You'll be given the tools to know what you can up-level in order to create an environment in which you will thrive, decrease stress, boost your energy, power up your immune system, and combat inflammation. First, we will help you identify your inflammation type. Then, we will find a diet plan that works best for you. And finally, we will help you identify the three nonnegotiable lifestyle shifts you need to make TODAY to stop inflammation from wreaking havoc on your life. When you reduce certain stressors and toxins in your life, you give your body the ability to build up energy to heal itself and do what it's supposed to do daily: balance hormones, regulate neurotransmitters, and so forth. Once your body has those internal energy reserves boosted, since it is now more able to keep your body healthy, it will be able to handle certain stressors that come its way, like that favorite spa-night-in face mask or your aunt's famous decadent pecan pie at Thanksgiving. Living an anti-inflammatory life isn't about being "perfect," adhering to a strict diet, staying inside to hide from any pollution, and strictly using organic products. An anti-inflammatory life the Maggie Berghoff Way is about taking ownership over the small choices and recognizing how every single one adds up, and consciously choosing each day to do things that will help your internal body thrive, while opting to, for the most part, avoid those that will be harmful.

There are a number of offenders we *can't* control, such as exhaust from cars on the road or the quality of the air inside our workplace. We'll learn about those factors and, more importantly, learn about the factors we *can* control in order to get you feeling your best as soon as possible. You'll finish this book with the tools you need to make choices that will decrease your Total Toxic Burden, keep unnecessary inflammation from happening, and consequently minimize or reverse the frustrating, painful, and nagging symptoms you've been experiencing. You'll also understand more about your specific Total Toxic Burden, including risk factors you may be predisposed to and how to combat them.

This book can also help you "biohack" and hit optimal performance and energy to become the best you can be. You don't have to be a professional athlete to need optimal performance. You need it for those kids you run around with, that loved one who wants to hang out after a long day, that career you want to expand. You need it for your family members, the hobby you want to enjoy, and simply that life you want to live. Even if you haven't struggled with symptoms similar to the ones from my own story or been diagnosed with a disease, it's empowering to recognize that the small choices you make all add up to have an effect on your body, your health, and therefore your life. Addressing inflammation can lead to more restful sleep, clear and younger-looking skin, less pain, and fewer bellyaches. Knowledge is power, and knowing the shifts you can make in your diet, environment, mindset, and product choices can entirely change how you show up in your life.

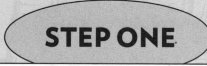

STEP ONE

YOUR INFLAMMATION TYPE

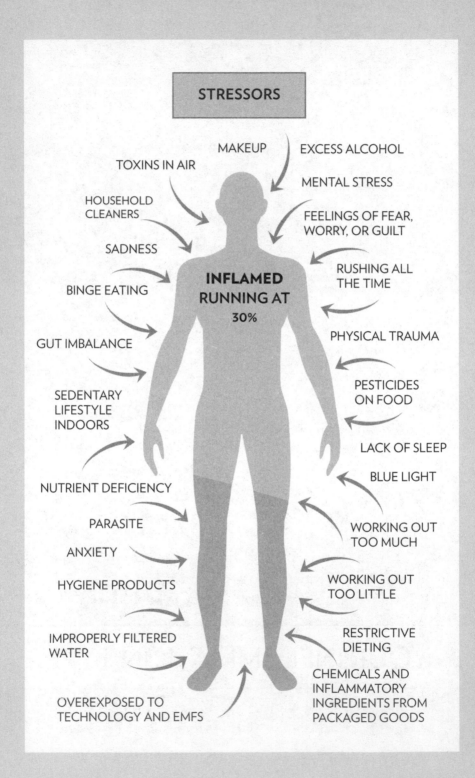

2

HOW TO IDENTIFY YOUR INFLAMMATION TYPE

"I MISS MY LIFE"

If you've ever thought to yourself, like so many of my clients have, "*I miss my life*," it's time to make a major shift. You don't have to struggle anymore—I am here for you.

Now that we understand inflammation and how it occurs, it's important to know your specific inflammation type. It may be caused by a host of different factors: your diet, environmental stressors, your genetics, and more. Knowing your specific inflammation type will help you navigate Step One of my program, where you identify which type (or types) are top priority for you and get clarity on what may be going on inside your body that is contributing to your symptoms. I encourage you to check out the chapters that relate to you based on your symptoms, conditions, or where you suspect you may be experiencing inflammation, so you can get some answers as to why certain conditions and symptoms occur and how you can begin to heal.

I would recommend working with a functional medicine practitioner or coach on your health, but also you absolutely can take your health into your own hands implementing the guidance in this book. Knowing your inflammation type, and the things that could be causing inflammation in your life, will completely change the way you feel day-to-day. You'll be able to simplify everything and know what to focus on to get better. It's also important to know that you may identify with multiple inflammation types, as inflammation in the body is widespread and can impact many different areas. This book will help you to know with more clarity what is going on, what the MAIN issues at hand are, and what to do next to resolve the inflammation in your body and heal. It can also help you to know what you may be predisposed to have, and what recommendations or chapters don't directly apply to you, so you can take this book at your pace and start feeling better sooner! All of this information will help you begin to take the right steps for *you*, which we'll cover in every inflammation type chapter. You can also visit maggieberghoff.com for book-related materials and support!

My team and I created a comprehensive quiz to help you determine your inflammation type. Be sure to head to the link and take the quiz right now before reading further. You can complete it on page 273 in this book, as well as at the link online, where you'll be given additional resources! In the following chapters, you will learn more about YOUR specific inflammation types and, in Steps Two and Three, learn customized tips to eat and live right!

Remember, you are a totally biochemically unique individual, and I do recommend that you get a deep assessment of your internal health via specialty laboratory data to guide your next steps beyond this book. However, taking the quiz to glean insights and following the guidance put forth in this book are your best immediate steps, and you'll learn tools for long term maintenance and vibrant living! This book alone will help you beyond anything you've ever tried before. You'll be given clarity, guidance, and hope. I believe in you; it's time for you to believe in you, too.

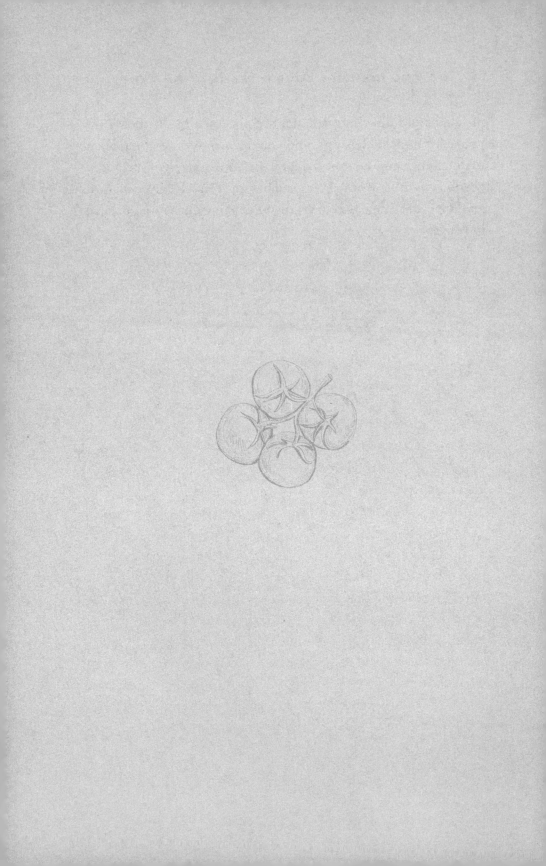

3

MUSCLE AND JOINT INFLAMMATION

Muscle and joint inflammation can keep you from living your life. Muscle aches don't help you to smile through your day, to run around with your kids or grandkids, to work all day without feeling the need to "couch it" all night. To live a vibrant and happy life, muscle and joint aches need to go. I'm here to help.

In this chapter, we'll survey the many instances of muscle and joint inflammation. As we unpack each common disease and symptom, we'll find that inflammation is at the root of each, which will help us better understand where the ROOT of the inflammation is influencing your health and how the reduction of this root cause can alleviate the symptoms of these aches and pains. Muscle and joint inflammation diseases include degenerative joint diseases such as rheumatoid arthritis and osteoarthritis, muscular dystrophy, the muscles within the lungs that can cause obstructive sleep apnea and other respiratory problems, and the buildup of plaque in our arteries, which is a muscular tube.

Beyond the expected diseases associated with muscles and joints, you may simply experience aches and pains, constant stiffness, and aching tightness in your muscles. Those who work out lifting heavy weights, or enjoy long-distance biking, swimming, or running, also may experience a lot of joint and muscle inflammation. If so, this chapter is definitely for you.

JOINT INFLAMMATION

According to the Centers for Disease Control and Prevention (CDC), in 2019, "In the United States, 23% of all adults, or more than 54 million people, have arthritis. It is a leading cause of work disability due to the pains and aches. The annual direct medical costs are at least $140 billion."[1] Simply put, arthritis refers to the inflammation of the joints that results in stiffness, soreness, and pain. The three most common types of arthritis are rheumatoid arthritis, osteoarthritis, and psoriatic arthritis (which affects both the skin and the joints).

QUICK CHECKLIST

You may have joint inflammation if:

❏ You experience swelling around one or multiple joints.
❏ You experience joint pain.
❏ Your joint function has become impaired, making it hard to do what you love to do or need to do.
❏ Your joint becomes stiff, or the range of motion is impaired.

We often think of arthritis as more probable with age, but there's a risk for joint inflammation at any age as the result of exceeding the body's Total Toxic Burden. I once worked with a recent college graduate named Austin who had just scored a great job in downtown Chicago. He was in his early twenties and in great physical shape . . . but woke up every morning feeling like an eighty-year-old man. The joint inflammation, aches, and pains were more than he could handle. Additionally, his hair was starting to fall out, and premature balding was not on his list of top ten things to experience right out of college.

As we began to work together and look beneath the surface, I learned that he was struggling with stress from his job. His dream was to start his own company, so he wasn't sure he should have been heading to a corporate office every day. Additionally, the social culture at the job included happy hours with bar food, shots, and cocktails—a few more nights every week than he'd like to admit to! He usually ate healthy, but felt he had to participate since he was the new guy at work and wanted to fit in with his coworkers. I get that. I do.

Now, Austin had never received any formal diagnosis for his aches and pains. But that didn't make them any less real, and he didn't know why he was experiencing them or how to fix them, which we addressed. Again, he wasn't downing fast food every day, drinking in huge excess, or lying on the couch eating potato chips from day to night. He was active! He was successful, fit, and looked "healthy." By all the standard measures! He was already doing fairly great things for his health, such as eating whole foods, filtering his water, and taking organic supplementations, and yet something was missing. His inflammation was the most severe in the morning, but we began to make changes for the entire day to reduce the inflammation as a whole and truly allow the body to heal itself from the inside out. We first needed to take a look at all his symptoms to determine if in fact we were dealing with joint inflammation as the primary concern.

His top symptoms were: joint pain every day, so much that it hurt him to stand up in the morning. He also complained about thinning hair, bloating, and digestive pain.

After looking over Austin's intake, it was clear that joint inflammation was his primary inflammation type. It was impacting his life in a major way, affecting his ability to work out, feel healthy, and sustain energy at work.

First, we focused on food. We added a lot more variety into his diet because he had been repeating many of the same food items, which was causing nutrient deficiencies, food intolerance, and health complications. All these things had led to even MORE inflammation and complications. Every time he was eating something his body couldn't tolerate, it was like he was pouring gas on the fire and making his inflammation worse.

We reduced any and all toxins in his downtown apartment as much as possible—cleaning his air with an air purifier, decreasing bright lights after sunset, and getting him a high-quality water filtration system to prevent heavy metals or bacteria from entering his body through water. After some tests, it was determined that there had been some bacteria in his gut, so we also addressed ridding his gut of the harmful bacteria, then rebuilding and repopulating his gut lining with healthy bacteria.

Once he was ready, we also implemented a full detoxification protocol to release his body of heavy metals, clean out his organs, and prime his body to accept more nutrients and to heal. Head to toe we addressed every system, every organ. We didn't just look at his joints, we looked at his gut health, nutrient levels, gallbladder, heavy metals, even the actual room he sleeps in—the works. The body is all connected, and improving these areas as well as his physical environment allows the body to heal in full.

I also helped Austin to alleviate stress, implementing calming tactics to help him stay out of his sympathetic nervous system, which, when elevated, chronically contributes to imbalances in the body and heightened inflammatory states. In other words, I helped him learn how to give himself a chill pill whenever he needed it! This helps more than you could imagine.

So, what happened?

After these changes, his aches and pains went away completely! No joke. It was almost as if he waved a magic wand over every icky thing he was experiencing, and vamoosh—back to normal. The bloating, the stress, the fatigue, all gone. Not only did the symptoms go away, but a new and even better "Austin" arose. He felt more inspired, positive, and fulfilled. So much so that he ended up quitting his corporate job and starting that new business during our time together. Without the aches and pains holding him back, he was able to live fully.

For detailed recommendations on how you can change your life and diet if you're experiencing joint pain, go to page 233.

RHEUMATOID ARTHRITIS

Rheumatoid arthritis (RA) is an autoimmune disease in which the body attacks its own healthy tissue, which certainly explains the aches and pains. So, instead of your body working in unison like it's supposed to, your immune system mistakes its own healthy tissue as the enemy and attacks it. Not good. This leads to the erosion of the healthy tissue, which makes joints feel chronically stiff, painful, and achy. There may be some swelling, too.

Rheumatoid arthritis can affect people in different areas, including the joints, the skin, the lungs, the eyes, and more. As with many autoimmune diseases, fatigue or constant feelings of sleepiness can be a symptom, because the body is spending all its energy trying to keep itself functioning while also trying to decrease the chaotic "war" going on inside. The body is under attack consistently—like a war that never ends—and, as a result, many people with autoimmune disease or symptoms of pain will begin to experience other symptoms as well. This is because the body is lacking the energy it would need to do other things it needs to do: digest your food, balance your hormones, or help you get a good night's rest and sleep soundly. Over time, the immune system's attack on the tissues around the joints can lead to bone deformation and loss of function. RA is considered to be chronic, or "incurable," by the conventional medical model.

QUICK CHECKLIST

You may have rheumatoid arthritis if:

- ❏ You have joint stiffness, especially first thing in the morning or after periods of inactivity.
- ❏ Joints are sore and swollen.
- ❏ Joints feel warm or hot to the touch.
- ❏ Joints appear red.
- ❏ In addition to these joint symptoms, you commonly feel sleepy and fatigued.

According to the *Journal of Inflammation*, "Traditionally, the standard treatment for rheumatoid arthritis has been to use a non-steroidal anti-inflammatory drug (NSAID), such as aspirin."[2] Inflammation is at the root of the pain, stiffness, and eventual bone and joint degradation of rheumatoid arthritis. It's true that an anti-inflammatory drug can reduce inflammation, but if we never resolve WHY the inflammation is happening in the first place, you'll be chasing symptoms and lab values forever . . . without ever truly being able to heal. Leak in the fridge, remember? So, instead of covering up the symptom with medication, I highly encourage you to seek out answers as to why the inflammation is happening in the first place. Where is it coming from? Why does your body not have the energy to heal itself? What is going on inside your body, mind, and life that is keeping you from fully feeling your best? Your aches and pains may absolutely be curable, but in order for that to be your truth, you must first identify why the inflammation is there. When the doctors can't help you, it's time to take matters into your own hands. Obviously, what you've been trying to do to heal hasn't worked, so let's dig deeper. Only YOU care enough about you to get well again. So, I ask you . . . where could your triggers be coming from?

I recently worked with a client named Jeanine who was seventy-six years old. She came to me because, simply put, she didn't want to *feel* old. She wanted to still be able to have an active lifestyle and work out, to visit her son and daughter-in-law and go canoeing with them, hike and bike frequently, and tend to her garden without any pain. However, she was struggling with rheumatoid arthritis, insulin sensitivity, insomnia, dizziness, and anxiety. She was on injection medications and other medicines to manage her pain and inflammation, as well as to help her go to sleep at night. As we'll soon learn about rheumatoid arthritis, it's considered an autoimmune disease and many doctors believe and tell their patients that there isn't a cure for it—and, therefore, it's something they'll have forever.

Jeanine believed that it was possible to live a life without the tremendous and exhausting pain in her joints that was robbing her of her ability to do all the activities she loved, so we worked together to get her life back. Before coming to me, she had been relying on heavy sleep medications for the past eighteen years to help her fall asleep at night. She was struggling to determine what "diet" to try to help her symptoms—which foods to eat more of? Which to avoid? She was doing all the "right things," it seemed, and yet she was left in pain and frustration day after day. Even pharmaceutical medications that were meant to alleviate her symptoms did little to help, and she was beginning to lose hope.

After working together, not only was she able to fall asleep swiftly and stay asleep throughout the night without any sleep medications, but she was able to greatly reduce the number of medications she took for her rheumatoid arthritis. This helped her to even complete part of a triathlon with her son and daughter-in-law without pain and swelling afterward or the need for medications! She felt as young as she had hoped to feel. She no longer felt like the arthritis was holding her back. Because, simply, it wasn't anymore!

Let's get you these results, too!

OSTEOARTHRITIS

Osteoarthritis develops when the cartilage that is supposed to act as a cushion between the bones wears down over time. The conventional medical community says that this wearing down of the cartilage happens either from the mechanical wear and tear of "overuse," or from an incident of joint trauma. So, if you were once an athlete and frequently used certain joints, leading to "wear and tear," that could be considered "a risk" in the conventional medical community—or, if there was any type of injury to the joint, that, too, could be an identifiable cause. Without the cartilage cushioning between the joints, painful abrasion between the bones happens . . . which is exactly what you feel! The pain, the aches, and the swelling arise. Osteoarthritis most commonly affects people in the areas of the hands, knees, hips, and spine.

Symptoms of osteoarthritis are quite similar to the symptoms of rheumatoid arthritis: swelling, stiffness, a general loss of flexibility in the affected joints, and tenderness or a bit of pain. To determine whether you have osteoarthritis, doctors will either conduct a blood test to make sure it isn't another disease (like rheumatoid arthritis) or do a joint fluid analysis, where they draw fluid via a needle from one of your affected joints.

QUICK CHECKLIST

You may have osteoarthritis if:

❏ You're experiencing swelling in your joints that has increased slowly throughout the years. Because osteoarthritis is caused by a gradual wear and tear, this pain and these symptoms increase incrementally.

❏ Your joints are stiff or you experience a general loss of flexibility.

❏ There is tenderness or a bit of pain in your joints.

Now, historically osteoarthritis has been thought to be *non*inflammatory, differing from rheumatoid arthritis, which is very much an *inflammatory* degenerative joint disease. However, it's been found that joint inflammation actually does play a role in developing osteoarthritis.

Research from the journal *Arthritis & Rheumatology* found that there are elevated levels of inflammatory plasma proteins in both the blood and the synovial (joint) fluids of patients with osteoarthritis.[3] Put very simply: *those with osteoarthritis have inflammation.* And the inflammation does not occur solely as a result of the wear and tear of the cartilage as you may expect.

It was actually found that the inflammation had been present in joints with osteoarthritis *before* the physical development of osteoarthritis. According to the American College of Rheumatology's classification criteria of osteoarthritis, there must be either "bony enlargement" or "osteophyte formation" on the joint.[4] This means that you have to already have inflammation and irregular bone formation in order for the doctors to diagnose you. In other words, when the damage is already done, they'll finally start some sort of treatment to help you. It's so backward. If inflammation was found in patients *before* the presence or development of irregular bone formation, and we'd just focus on reducing a person's inflammation, the "disease" would never have the opportunity to happen in the first place! We could save endless healthcare dollars. We could prevent endless people from suffering through life. We could create a more uplifting and positive world full of people who feel amazing, inside and out. So frustrating.

The study went on to report that this chronic inflammation contributes to all degenerative joint diseases. The inflammation may have initially happened as the result of joint trauma—acute inflammation that became chronic. However it occurred, the vicious cycle of local tissue damage, inflammation, and repair happens again and again. Over time, this chronic inflammation causes osteoarthritis. Even though it's frustrating that this could have been prevented, it happened. You're here now and you're in pain. But just know that there is hope and you can absolutely thrive again!

Although osteoarthritis is not an autoimmune disorder, I help clients with osteoarthritis in the same way I help them with rheumatoid arthritis . . . and in the same way I help clients with any type of ache, pain, "incurable condition," disease, you name it! We look at all the stressors in their life, take stock of their Total Toxic Burden, and see where we can alleviate the stressors on the body. Aches and pains can show up as a myriad of different diagnoses that a conventional doctor may give you—but at the heart they're *each* able to be allevi ated with a few changes that will help your body heal. You get to choose from this moment on: Will you continue to live life like this? Or, will you implement the methods within this book and be forever changed? I hope and pray you choose the latter! You in?!

JOINT INFLAMMATION CAUSED BY MICROBIOTA IN THE GUT

Now, let's talk about the gut again! The deeper assessment of inflammation is holistic, and there are far more connections than you'd initially think between different systems within the body, which is why we'll get quite friendly with the inner work ings of your gut throughout this book! Case in point: there's research that has found that the gut can cause that aching, swell ing inflammation in the joints.

Specifically, a change in "microbiota composition" is linked to joint disease activity. Microbiota are simply the microorgan isms that live inside your gut. There are both good bacteria and, well, *bad* bacteria, and whenever a client takes a test that points to problems in the gut (such as with Austin), we work to remove the bad bacteria and promote more of the good bacteria within the gut lining. Microbiota can change their composition based on your diet and can also change if you take antibiotics because you get sick or have an infection.

Researchers found that microscopic gut inflammation was observed in 50% of patients with arthritis and has been linked to disease activity, underscoring the effects of gut inflamma tion in arthritis.[5] In other words, if something is off in the gut that causes it to become inflamed, your body may become more susceptible to muscle and joint pains.

The research found that changes to the microbiota in the gut, or dysbiosis (which is a microbial imbalance), contribute to the development of various forms of inflammatory arthritis. These bad boys do the inflammation work we know so well in the joints—specifically, the synovial joints, which are any joints that allow movement. These include ball-and-socket joints (your shoulders), hinge joints (your knees), pivot joints (in the vertebrae of your neck), condyloid joints (in your wrist), and saddle joints (your thumb and shoulder).

So, when your gut health is not on point, it deeply affects other areas of your body outside of the gut. The research found that there is indeed a "close association between the composition of the microbiota and inflammatory diseases." The gut is a very important area to consider when working with clients who are experiencing joint inflammation or muscle pains. It's absolutely not the final answer, though. Remember, we must ask: Why is the gut microbiome out of balance? What caused that? Then, go deeper and deeper into the investigation of the top core stressors or factors that must be addressed in each individual's life. That's why many of my clients and peers refer to me as a "health detective," because I'm essentially doing deep detective work to determine how to best reduce certain stressors in the client's life, optimize the internal biochemistry, and allow the body to heal! Step aside, Nancy Drew!

For more detailed help if you have joint inflammation caused by microbiota, go to page 233.

MUSCLE INFLAMMATION

With muscle inflammation, you may feel sore all the time, aching, or tight in your muscles. It feels like a chronic pain you simply may feel that you've "always had." It doesn't seem directly correlated to anything really—just a constant nagging, aching pain.

You may have muscle inflammation if:

❑ You feel sore, achy, and stiff.

❑ You have to take days off from exercise due to soreness after a workout.

❑ After a day of activity or walking a lot, you feel increased aches and pains.

FIBROMYALGIA

Another autoimmune disease that causes pain in your muscles and bones is fibromyalgia. It often coexists with chronic pain syndrome, and can also cause fatigue, general areas of tenderness on your body, and cognitive disruption. In fibromyalgia, the brain and its nerves misread normal pain signals, creating a constant, dull ache that lasts for months. Even just a light press against one region of the body can feel painful when you have fibromyalgia—in fact, it can be diagnosed by a doctor pressing lightly against the body's eighteen trigger points (such as the tops of the shoulders, knees, and upper chest). If eleven of those eighteen trigger points experience pain, a fibromyalgia diagnosis is likely.[6]

You may have fibromyalgia if:

❑ You experience fatigue and heavy brain fog that disrupts your cognitive function.

❏ You're experiencing pain throughout your body, specifically within the muscles. It may feel like a "tender pain" as opposed to a sharp pain.

❏ You have problems with sleeping well, thwarted memory, and irritable mood as a result of the pain.

The symptoms can be quite extensive—dry eyes, depression, anxiety, symptoms similar to irritable bowel syndrome (IBS), trouble sleeping, muscle spasms, and bladder problems. There is also a symptom colloquially called "fibro fog," which is another term for the brain fog and a general sense of exhaustion and confusion that are present. Problems with memory may result.

CHRONIC PAIN SYNDROME

Then there's chronic pain syndrome, which is yet again marked by constant and chronic aches and pains: lower-back pain, joint pain, muscle aches, headaches, and the occasional jolt of sharper pain. You may notice a trend here! Chronic pain syndrome often begins with an acute initial injury or illness, which then leads to chronic pain that continues for three to six months or longer, and can lead to fatigue, trouble sleeping, and mood changes, including depression and irritability. Here's the catch, though. Many people have acute injuries or illnesses in their life but do not end up suffering from chronic pain. It's not a surefire symptom of experiencing an injury or illness at one point in your life. Your body is supposed to regenerate and heal! So, what makes these men and women who bounce back easily so different? Why is it that some bodies DO develop long-term pain and symptoms? Well, it boils down to their internal and external health, thoughts, and lifestyle. Typically, these clients who experience more lasting pains have other inflammatory stressors going on in their lives that make them more susceptible to experiencing chronic pain. When we address those stressors, strengthen the body's internal chemistry, and boost the immune system, we can make tremendous progress toward alleviating chronic pain!

QUICK CHECKLIST

You may have chronic pain syndrome if:

- ❏ You experience consistent pain that lasts weeks, months, and even years.
- ❏ The pain feels like a "burning" or a tingly, pins-and-needles sensation.
- ❏ The pain is classified as joint or muscle pain. It can also appear as lower-back pain and constant headaches.
- ❏ The pain contributes to insomnia and trouble sleeping, frequent fatigue, depression, and anxiety.

Here's the good news: regardless of the specific type of disease or syndrome that's making every day and every night challenging, achy, painful, and exhausting, there may be a way to fix it. "Incurable," "chronic," "lifelong"—these words and diagnoses may not have to be a part of your story—let's remove them, shall we? You have control over the next step in your life. Your body CAN heal itself. I'm here to help and am sending all the positive vibes your way right now! Can you feel it?

For detailed nutrition and lifestyle tips tailored for you, go to page 233!

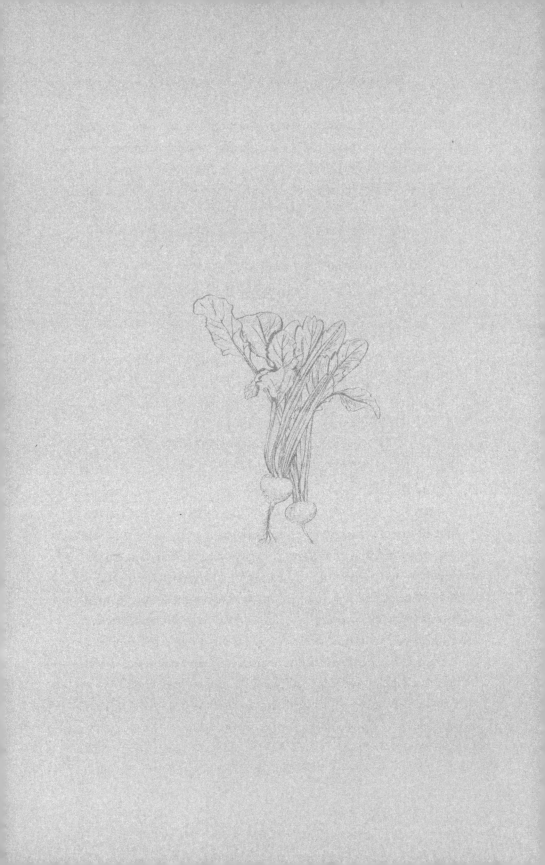

4

HORMONAL AND THYROID INFLAMMATION

When I was younger, I was constantly freezing. It could be a hot summer day and everyone else would be in spaghetti straps and shorts, and I'd be sporting a big sweater and warm fuzzy socks. Since my mom had attended the Cancer Treatment Centers of America in her quest to heal herself and therefore had an understanding of functional medicine, she always suspected that my thyroid was underactive because of my constant state of the shivers.

She even took me to the doctor on multiple occasions throughout my teenage years to see if I had an underactive thyroid or abnormal hormone levels, but all my labs consistently would come back "normal." Nothing showed up in the conventional medicine model. Looking back now, I can't believe that those doctors ignored my symptoms because their printed lab report didn't have a bolded "H" or "L" next to my levels. They never investigated deeper, despite my constant symptoms of feeling cold and tired, and—all the more concerning—the fact that I didn't even have cycles! I didn't have my first menstrual cycle until I was eighteen years old, and it only started when I finally gave in to taking the birth control pills my doctors had been wanting me to get on for years in an attempt to medically induce my cycle. I had all of these wonky symptoms, but they weren't showing up in any evidence-based way, so the doctors didn't do anything about them . . . until, of course, my body crashed at age twenty-four. Even then, there were no answers to fix my body. All I got from my doctors was, "There's nothing we can do about this," and "Here, take these medications . . . you'll need them for the rest of your life."

In the conventional model of medicine, an internal imbalance usually isn't identifiable from lab results until it's too late and the body already has a full-blown disease resulting from the imbalance, such as cancer or, in my case, Hashimoto's disease, prediabetes, and PCOS (polycystic ovarian syndrome) as it relates to the thyroid and hormones. People need help with symptoms that often go unnoticed and are essentially ignored until something happens that is so severe that a doctor can finally identify it with a lab value and then prescribe a pharmaceutical medication to "fix" that lab value, find a cancer they can identify and cut out, or find a heart disease they can go in and patch up. This needs to change.

AN INTRODUCTION TO YOUR THYROID AND HORMONES

Here is a quick background on the endocrine system: your body has many hormones that work together to do the things we need the body to do—produce melatonin to fall asleep at night, respond to stress (whether it's a true fight-or-flight situation because a black bear just poked its head from around the tree in the woods on your camping trip, or you're simply stressed about work), regulate fertility and your menstrual cycles, manage blood sugar so you don't feel like you're going to pass out if you haven't eaten lately. Hormones are responsible for all of that and so much more! Go team!

An important part of the endocrine system is the thyroid: a butterfly-shaped gland that sits in your throat, right by your voice box and your trachea. Your thyroid is responsible for releasing hormones that keep your body in "homeostasis," which essentially means "balanced," so that cells can function properly and everything can work in business as usual. Your thyroid regulates body temperature (hence, my fuzzy socks all summer long when mine was underactive), skin moisture, energy, mood, brain development, digestion, and much, much more. It's quite important! We rely on the thyroid to keep releasing hormones properly so that our body can stay in homeostasis. Otherwise, many wonky symptoms start to show up . . . like, for me, the absence of menstrual cycles, bloating, and more.

The most common symptoms I see in clients with any type of hormonal imbalance or issue with the thyroid include painful or irregular menstrual cycles, depression, anxiety, weight gain, hair thinning or falling out, cold all the time, bloating, and food cravings. If you experience any of these—or suspect or have received a doctor's diagnosis for hormonal imbalance, infertility, hypothyroidism, an overactive thyroid, or any condition related to your hormones or thyroid—this chapter is for you.

QUICK CHECKLIST

You may have hormone and thyroid inflammation if:

- ❏ You're cold all the time—sometimes freezing even in the middle of summer.
- ❏ You're gaining weight. You can't lose weight. If you do lose weight, it comes back so easily—what

took months to come off can come back on in a
day or so.

❑ You may have hair growing where you wish it
wouldn't, like your chin.

❑ You're anxious or depressed, so much that
it's impacting your lifestyle and personal
relationships. You don't feel like yourself anymore
and you'd rather hide away at home than go out.

❑ You get bloated or have constipation. It can look
like you're several months pregnant all the time.

❑ You have irregular menstrual cycles. Maybe you
don't have any at all and laugh it off as "lucky," or
you have a lot of painful and frustrating symptoms
around your cycles. Maybe they're just super
random and each month is different.

❑ You can't get pregnant and infertility is becoming
a concern.

❑ You have cravings for sugar/carbs. You feel like
you're always hungry or wanting sugars and carbs.

❑ You have dry or oily skin.

❑ You're so very tired. You get home from work, hit
the couch, and are there for the evening.

❑ The brain fog is real. You just feel "off" and aren't
as "sharp" as you used to be. Things are foggy.

UNDERACTIVE THYROID OR HYPOTHYROIDISM

An underactive thyroid simply means your thyroid doesn't
produce or release enough of the hormones that it needs to in
order to keep your body functioning properly. As a result, symptoms such as constantly being cold, weight gain, depression, and

fatigue may occur. Over time, hypothyroidism can lead to more serious conditions, such as infertility, heart disease, obesity, and joint pain. Specifically, hypothyroidism means that the thyroid isn't releasing two important hormones: T3, which affects body temperature, heart rate, and your metabolism, and T4, which plays a role in digestion, the maintenance of the bones, the heart function, the muscles, and brain development.

T3 is the function that is most often seen as low and contributes to the majority of the symptoms that a client notices. It's the active form of thyroid in the body. Hypothyroidism can be a low level in any of these markers, which is why it's important to have your practitioner check, at the very minimum, a TSH, T4, T3, and thyroid antibodies when looking into thyroid health. Many doctors will only check a TSH level, which is a poor indicator of thyroid health because TSH may be completely "normal" on a lab test, but the level of T4 or T3 could be low.

QUICK CHECKLIST

You may have hypothyroidism if:

- ❏ You're frequently cold (do fuzzy socks year-round ring a bell?).
- ❏ You tend to be more sluggish and fatigued, regardless of how much rest you get.
- ❏ You're experiencing symptoms of depression— you just want to be alone all the time and you feel a baseline of sadness, which isn't like you.
- ❏ Weight gain is getting really annoying. You're gaining weight "out of nowhere" and it's noticeable. You used to be able to lose weight with ease, and now it's nearly impossible to lose or to keep it off once you do lose.

❑ Your eating habits are getting out of control. You
never feel satisfied or full and are always wanting
more.

❑ Your menstrual cycles are irregular and are, more
often than not, pretty much absent. You can go
months, even years, without having a period.

HASHIMOTO'S THYROIDITIS

One cause of thyroid complications that often goes undiagnosed
is called Hashimoto's disease, which is an autoimmune disorder
in which the body's immune system begins to attack the thyroid.
Since it's under attack, the thyroid can't produce or release the
hormones that it needs to. One of the main causes of Hashimoto's is stress, but not just mental stress. When I refer to "stress,"
I'm referring to anything that places stress on the body and its
internal biochemistry. That can be mental stress, yes, but also
stress from your food choices, the toxins in your environment, a
sedentary lifestyle, and more.

One indicator that you may have Hashimoto's is swelling
in your thyroid—but you can have Hashimoto's with no swelling at all. It may be sore to the touch and look swollen from the
front of your neck. This may cause infertility, problems with
your menstrual cycle, and pregnancy complications, as well as
the symptoms of hypothyroidism we discussed above: bloating,
weight gain or loss, anxiety or depression, fatigue, brain fog,
thinning hair, dry skin, and more.

If you suspect Hashimoto's disease, you will need a full
thyroid panel including thyroid antibodies to assess if your
thyroid is attacking itself. And if you do test positive for
Hashimoto's or hypothyroidism, your doctor may prescribe a
daily thyroid pill in order to give the body the thyroid hormones

it needs to function fully. However, this pill is not the solution to healing the thyroid—it simply gives the thyroid the hormones that it needs from an outside source. Sometimes the medication can even make things worse, because the body then thinks it has plenty of thyroid hormones, so shuts down its own processes of producing them. That said, it can help bridge the gap between feeling better right now and actually reversing and healing the thyroid condition long-term. Ultimately, it's essential to know that you must identify *why* the thyroid is under attack and why it's underperforming in order to ever have a shot at healing it for good and thus stopping medications. Don't let your thyroid gland get lazy and dependent on a pill you're popping! Help it to do what it's supposed to do again.

Once you identify and address the root causes, and combat inflammation in the body (thus changing the internal environment), the thyroid will again be able to produce and release hormones as it's supposed to, and you can live a life free of symptoms or complications.

QUICK CHECKLIST

You may have Hashimoto's disease if:

- ❏ You are experiencing visible swelling on the front of your throat where your thyroid gland is located.
- ❏ You have been gaining weight no matter what you do—AND it almost seems like the more you work out and try to lose, the more you gain!
- ❏ You are sluggish and fatigued and get cold easily (or struggle to warm up)—you hate it . . . a human popsicle, you could say.
- ❏ Your skin and hair are dry or rough, no matter how many deep-conditioning treatments you use or

how many lotions you try. I mean, you've lathered your body in coconut oil at night and still don't have the silky-smooth skin you envy. Even that lip balm that swears it's the ONE lip balm that will finally heal your lips, no luck for you.

❏ You notice more hair than usual in the drain after your showers. You never used to lose hair, and it's freaking you out.

❏ You're experiencing constipation. You've tried it all—drinks, pills, laxatives, gut detox teas—and nothing works except to cause you horrible cramping and pain, maybe some diarrhea. You can go days or even weeks without pooping.

❏ You're nodding asleep in meetings or class even though you slept eight-plus hours. You're straining to keep your eyes open, squinting to type and read as your eyes start to roll back.

I was diagnosed with Hashimoto's when my thyroid levels were finally out of balance enough to show up in my lab values as a red flag. However, it's clear that my body had thyroid abnormalities and underperformance long before this "diagnosis" or "abnormal" lab value. After healing my body through the means you'll discover in this book, I no longer experience any of the symptoms of hypothyroidism, and I'm off thyroid medication completely. If you have an underactive thyroid or Hashimoto's, I urge you to ask more questions as to why your thyroid may be out of balance, and not simply blame "genetics" or some other cause. Yes, my mom has hypothyroidism. Yes, my grandmother has hypothyroidism. But you know what? That doesn't have to be a part of my story, and it isn't anymore. Know that there is almost always a way to heal your thyroid for good!

OVERACTIVE THYROID OR HYPERTHYROIDISM

Rather than producing too few hormones as in hypothyroidism, an overactive thyroid produces *too many*. And, because a perfectly balanced and functioning body requires homeostasis, too many hormones isn't good, either. We need an internal balance—so too much or too little won't do!

Now, when you think of an overactive thyroid, the symptoms oftentimes (but not always) mirror the symptoms of an underactive thyroid, but on the inverse. Think through the opposites. Rather than constantly being fatigued, someone with an overactive thyroid typically has abounding energy—an uncomfortable amount! They may experience tremors or shakes (like you'd experience if you drank too many espresso shots), nonstop sweating and constantly feeling hot, insomnia, more frequent bowel movements, weight loss, hair loss, irritability, and constant hunger. An overactive thyroid can also lead to bulging eyeballs or the inability to close your eyes because of swelling in the eye tissues.

Then, similar to hypothyroidism, someone with hyperthyroidism may also have irregular or painful cycles. Cycles are often impacted in some way by an imbalance in thyroid hormone production.

QUICK CHECKLIST

You may have hyperthyroidism or Graves' disease if:

❏ You're hot in the middle of a Chicago winter.

❏ You sleep four hours a night if you're lucky.

❏ You're sweating way more than you'd like to admit . . . and have to cart around extra deodorant as a result.

❏ No matter how much you eat or how sedentary your lifestyle is, you're shedding pounds left and right and it scares you.

❏ You lie awake at night, wired, counting sheep but unable to get adequate sleep.

❏ You feel a pulsing heartbeat almost in your head all the time.

❏ You feel anxious and shaky, and your thoughts are running wild.

❏ Your stools are loose and you're running to the bathroom often.

GRAVES' DISEASE

Graves' disease is another autoimmune disorder in which the immune system attacks the thyroid, but this attack causes the thyroid to produce far *more* hormones than your body needs. Your immune system's antibodies actually mimic thyroid-stimulating hormones, so your thyroid doesn't know how to turn off. To understand this, think back to a time when you stepped outside into a snowstorm. Almost instantly, you started to shiver as your body got colder from the outside temperature. To return your body to homeostasis, your hypothalamus sent these thyroid-stimulating hormones to the thyroid to tell it to warm you up. It's your body's way of turning on its internal fireplace or heater.

In Graves' disease, the hypothalamus isn't the one sending the signals. Rather, it's the antibodies sent by your immune system *pretending to be the hormones*, and they put on a good show—like, Oscar worthy! The thyroid doesn't know it needs to stop because it perceives the antibodies as the stimulating hormones. So it keeps producing more hormones than it needs to. It doesn't know it's doing anything wrong, even though the hypothalamus is yelling to please, please stop because we're burning up here!

The only ways that Graves' can be "cured" are by targeting the thyroid with antithyroid medications or the removal of part or all of the thyroid gland. However, the immune system doesn't stop producing these impostor antibodies despite these treatments, so they only work as a Band-Aid to the underlying problem. So we might as well target the underlying problem—that leak in the fridge.

Graves' disease and Hashimoto's thyroiditis can actually go hand in hand (in other words, you could have both or sway between the two), because they're both hormonal imbalances and autoimmune disorders. In fact, having one autoimmune disorder of any type can put you at risk for being diagnosed with another, too. Research from the *American Journal of Medicine* found that it's important to screen "for other autoimmune diagnoses if subjects with autoimmune thyroid disease present with new or nonspecific symptoms." Specifically, their study found that the frequency of having another autoimmune disorder was 9.67% in Graves' disease and 14.3% in Hashimoto's thyroiditis, and interestingly, the most common coexisting autoimmune disorder was rheumatoid arthritis.[1] These imbalances and disorders tend to have a domino effect when not dealt with properly.

The best way to take control of both and all autoimmune conditions is to remove the stressors that are causing the body to attack the thyroid. The body must return to homeostasis with the proper levels of hormones, and it can't do this unless some serious stressors are mediated.

SEX HORMONAL IMBALANCE

Other glands in your body that produce hormones aside from your thyroid are your ovaries, and a hormonal imbalance can be caused in the ovaries that leads to the overproduction or underproduction of certain sex hormones, such as progesterone, testosterone, and estrogen. The fluctuation of these hormones is actually normal over your lifetime—such as when you went through puberty, during pregnancy, breastfeeding, perimenopause (right before menopause), and menopause. The problem arises when these hormones become too imbalanced, or their imbalance is chronic.

QUICK CHECKLIST

You may have a sex hormonal imbalance if you experience:

- ❏ Mood swings from high to low, happy to sad
- ❏ A sense that your heart is beating out of your chest, or that it skips a beat (like when you've had one too many shots of espresso)
- ❏ Irritability—over pretty much anything
- ❏ Trouble concentrating; your brain feels foggy and you feel a general "blah" feeling and can't zone in on what you're supposed to be focusing on
- ❏ Irregular cycles—you may be the one bawling at the simplest things around "that time of the month," in bed all day from pain, super on edge, craving chocolate like no one else. You may even be the one who doesn't ever have a cycle at all. . . . When the doctor asks you when your last menstrual cycle was, you have NO clue—did I have a period this year?

POLYCYSTIC OVARIAN SYNDROME

One of the most common conditions that results from hormonal imbalances is polycystic ovarian syndrome, or PCOS. It's actually quite common—one in ten women between puberty and perimenopause will have it.[2] I, too, was diagnosed with it in my twenties. PCOS leads to symptoms such as irregular menstrual cycles, acne, thinning hair, and weight gain.

As with each of these hormonal conditions, there are medications you can be prescribed to help with the symptoms, but as we know, your best chance for healing yourself is to heal your stressors so the body can return to balance. The medications often do not "fix" the problem at all, and you'll struggle with the "diagnosis" year after year. I'd rather give you the tools and strategies to put your health into your own hands and actually reverse the problem and have PCOS go away completely than to give you a pill to just help with your symptoms.

QUICK CHECKLIST

You may have PCOS if:

- ❏ Aunt Flow comes to visit irregularly or not at all.
- ❏ You are struggling with fertility problems.
- ❏ Your skin tends to be oily and acne-prone, and your favorite skin cleanser isn't helping.
- ❏ Weight gain comes easily and weight loss is more difficult—but know that you *may* also be really thin! I was very thin despite my PCOS diagnosis until things got even worse, so don't feel that you have to fit the "overweight" category to have PCOS.

❑ You have excessive hair growth over your body and it's to the point that it's embarrassing.

LOW PROGESTERONE

There are two main female hormones: progesterone and estrogen—both of which are responsible for helping the body start menstruation. Specifically, progesterone is secreted after ovulation, whereas estrogen is secreted beforehand. Low levels of progesterone can cause symptoms such as irregular cycles, anxiety, depression, headaches or migraines—not to mention a challenge in helping your body get pregnant, if you're trying. Low progesterone can also lead to weight gain and mood swings.

QUICK CHECKLIST

You may have low progesterone if:

❑ You are struggling with infertility.
❑ You have frequent headaches or migraines.
❑ You have a tendency to experience anxiety or depression, in addition to mood swings.
❑ Your menstrual cycles are irregular.

HIGH TESTOSTERONE AND ESTROGEN

Another common imbalance I see frequently is high levels of testosterone and estrogen. Yes, the female body also produces testosterone! It's produced by the ovaries, and although we don't have as much testosterone as men do, it also plays a role in our reproductive processes. But if a hormonal imbalance occurs that causes higher levels of testosterone, there may be less frequent or heavy menstrual cycles and even the development of more body hair. High levels of testosterone actually occur frequently in polycystic ovarian syndrome.

High levels of estrogen also throw off a body's balance. During puberty and the early months of pregnancy, estrogen naturally rises. But if you aren't in either of these stages, the rise of estrogen can lead to icky symptoms, like weight gain, insomnia or fatigue, hair loss, headaches, and bloating.

I'm sure you can pick up on the trend here: whenever any hormone is off-balance, regardless of which hormone it is and whether the levels are too high or too low, symptoms occur that rob you of the energy, vitality, and general feelings of wellness that you deserve. While there are many medications that claim to "treat" each imbalance, the only way to truly restore your body's homeostasis is to reduce the stressors that cause the imbalances in the first place. The truth is, the medications rarely "treat" anything; they're just a Band-Aid to help cover up the symptoms. A balanced body has healthy menstrual cycles, a healthy weight, and isn't ridden by the uncomfortable and irritating symptoms that get in the way of your vibrant health! Your body knows how to produce, balance, and regulate hormones. It is far smarter than any pill prescribed. You simply need to fix the internal and external environment and reduce inflammatory stressors in order to allow your body to thrive!

WOMEN'S INFERTILITY

Infertility is another devastating side effect of a hormonal imbalance. Because my own specific area of expertise (and my own experience) is geared more toward women's health when speaking about hormone levels, I will cover women's infertility here, just as I covered women's sex hormones. Of course, infertility can also be a man's reality, so if you are a male and suspect infertility, I recommend scheduling an appointment with a functional medicine practitioner to confirm and create a treatment plan. Regardless, the inflammation cures and reduction of stressors within this book are likely to help, even for men. The techniques taught here are equally important in both males and females of all ages. Everyone can benefit from adding anti-inflammatory regimens into their routines!

Now, there is an entire host of reasons that infertility may occur. I specifically help clients who are experiencing infertility as a side effect of hormonal imbalances, or excessive stress or toxicities that cause chaos internally. When the body is in a fight-or-flight mode, it simply doesn't have the time or energy to continue its regular fertility and ovulation cycles. It halts the reproductive system (and other systems, such as digestion) to focus on the problem at hand and the corresponding stress. This also results in quite a chaotic internal state, which is no place to conceive or nourish a baby!

Infertility can also occur from PCOS, as we've learned. If the ovaries do not release an egg to be fertilized, conception won't occur. Hormonal imbalances can make it difficult for your body to be in the right balance to support a fetus or release an egg.

If you ever learned about the process of ovulation and a woman's menstrual cycles in school, you learned that there is a very specific, diligent, complex process that occurs to create an egg that makes it into the fallopian tube to meet with the sperm. It requires a perfect harmony of exact hormones and every part of the reproductive system working exactly as it should for the miracle of conception. To give your body the best chance at conceiving, your body's homeostasis must be at its most ideal state. Any stress or toxicities may prevent your body from getting pregnant.

In my case, I was told I was infertile and would never have a baby because I wasn't ovulating at all. My hormones simply didn't release an egg to be fertilized that could become a baby. My body was failing, I had PCOS and Hashimoto's, my toxicity levels were through the roof, and my sugar levels were all over the place. To make matters worse, my progesterone levels were really low, and my estrogen and testosterone levels were really high. The hormonal imbalance made it impossible for me to become pregnant—and I wasn't even ovulating, so there was no egg that could even be fertilized when my body was in this chaotic state.

If I had accepted my fate as it was given from the conventional medical model, I likely would not be the proud mother of three young and healthy little ones. You see, once I was able to rebalance my body, I became pregnant immediately (and naturally, without medical intervention). Despite being told I was infertile, I was able to restore balance within my body by making the necessary changes. I want this for you, too. With clients of mine who have struggled with getting pregnant, their body returned to balance once we handled food intolerances, levels of stress, and levels of inflammation in their environment—which could include their gut health, home environment, and even their mental state. Within months, they became pregnant after years of trying. It's near miraculous to see this happen, and it can totally happen for you, too.

However, I'm not a miracle worker—and I don't want you to think that I had some magical prescription that got them pregnant. It wasn't an expensive round of IVF. It wasn't injections I gave them daily to boost certain hormone levels. All I helped them to do was reinstate balance in the body so the body could do what it naturally wanted to do in the first place. Your body wants to heal. You see, these women didn't "have" infertility—their internal environment simply was not in the state to become pregnant due to the stressors and inflammation. Once we addressed those factors, the body was able to produce a healthy and natural pregnancy. There *is* hope for you—and your body is powerful beyond measure! As I always say, we just have to give it a helping hand.

For detailed nutrition and lifestyle tips tailored for you, go to page 233.

5

INFLAMMATION FROM SUGAR

'm going to just put it out there. Almost *everyone* in the world has sugar inflammation. Sugar is inflammatory, and most of you are consuming it even when you don't realize it. I'll explain what I mean later. So, no matter your core inflammation type, sugar inflammation is likely a secondary type and something to be addressed. It can also be a trigger for all the other inflammation types.

Now, let's talk about sugar in more detail. The average American consumes *far more* than the daily recommended allowance for sugar consumption.

With my own health decline, sugar didn't just contribute to my body swelling, it would even make my body feel sore to the touch. It was so weird. If I dug into a bag of chocolate-covered pretzels or downed a candy-covered ice cream treat, I would wake up the next day feeling as though the entire surface area of my skin were bruised. It would hurt to the touch from the inflammation, especially around my neck and face, but really everywhere. Granted, at times I would eat a LOT of sugar at once, bingeing out on it and usually with other "unhealthy" foods.

Now I can eat sugar and be totally fine—no swelling, no inflammation, no pain, no mood changes, no skin changes. I encourage you to eliminate it completely right now, but know that eventually your body will be able to compensate for the sugar inflammation and be just fine with enjoying it here and there!

There really is absolutely zero nutritional value in cane sugar and processed sugar. The most common symptoms I've seen sugar consumption lead to are acne, skin breakouts, anxiety, depression, gut bloating, swelling, and weight gain.

This chapter's intention is to fill you in on exactly what happens when the body consumes too much sugar, and how it can lead to less-than-ideal symptoms, such as high blood pressure, cravings, a growing waistline, a sugar addiction, and conditions such as prediabetes, diabetes, and insulin sensitivity. I know that removing sugar can sometimes be the last thing you want to do—especially if you have that favorite sugary latte or heavenly weekend dessert that you look forward to treating yourself to. But, by learning about how sugar can impact the body, I hope it helps you see sugar differently. This knowledge will help you empower yourself to reduce the number of toxins you expose your body to; and yes, too much sugar can be a toxin.

This chapter is also for anyone who finds themselves crashing energy-wise after eating a meal or who feels starving an hour after having breakfast. We'll break down the metabolic process in this chapter, too—so if losing or managing your weight is a goal this year, you'll also benefit from the pages ahead.

QUICK CHECKLIST

You may have sugar inflammation if:
- ❑ You're irritable and emotional.

❑ You have energy highs, then energy crashes.

❑ You have anxiety and problems focusing—like ADHD-type symptoms.

❑ You have acne as an adult.

HOW YOUR BODY BREAKS DOWN SUGAR

Time for a brief lesson: sugar contains both glucose and fructose. Fructose on its own does not contain any nutritional value. However, many fruits have high levels of fructose, and as you know, most people think of fruits as healthy. They are! It really comes down to the quantity or type of fruit consumed, when it's eaten, and how it's prepared. Whole fruit, such as an apple, is great to consume in moderation because it also has fiber and water, which allows the body to break it down slowly, and consequently metabolize fructose slowly. Fructose on its own (such as if you had a spoonful of pure high fructose corn syrup) must be sent to the liver, which will break it down into glycogen. Think of glycogen as your body's fuel tank. It's energy waiting to be used for any sudden and strenuous burst of activity.

However, your body can store only so much glycogen. When the tank is full, it won't accept any more—just like when your car is full at the gas station, the pump stops. It won't even continue the faucet of fuel. Full means full. If you're still consuming more fructose than you need to, your liver will halt the production of glycogen, and instead turn the extra fructose into fat.

Then there's glucose—which *does* have some nutritional value—in moderation (and the key word is moderation!). Glucose is found in proteins such as fish, meat, and cheese, in fats such as avocados and butter, and in starches and whole grains.

We consume glucose in carbohydrates, too. Every time you eat a bowl of pasta or a slice of bread, you're consuming glucose.

When the body metabolizes glucose, the pancreas is signaled to make insulin, a hormone with one sole responsibility: to regulate glucose in the bloodstream. Insulin carries the glucose to one of three cells—liver, muscle, or fat cells—during the metabolic process. Insulin also carries fructose, but fructose doesn't command insulin from the pancreas in quite the same way that glucose does.

Think of insulin as a hotel keeper. It has the keys to all the different "rooms"—the liver cells, muscle cells, and fat cells. It carries the glucose or fructose to be deposited into these cells by connecting to each cell's insulin receptor and "unlocking" the cell, then escorting the glucose inside.

A problem arises when you consume too much glucose. The liver, muscle, and fat cells will try to store it, but if they can't because they're crammed full, the glucose will be deposited back into the bloodstream, causing a spike in blood sugar. The glucose will have nowhere to go, so it runs rampant causing trouble without a "home."

I also like to think of it this way. Imagine your body as a machine. It needs fuel in order to work properly and have all its systems working. Now, if we dump a bunch of sticky and gooey liquid (ahem . . . sugar) into that machine, it's going to clog up the system. Some of the gears may get sticky and stop working. Other parts of the machine will malfunction, too. And . . . you now have a broken machine.

This metaphor is what sugar does to your body! On the flip side, if you give the machine the nourishing fluid it needs (I'm talking about the high-quality whole foods that are full of nutrients and antioxidants), then the machine will be able to perform at its best every day. That's what I want for you: to fuel your body in a way that allows it to be its very best. And that means daily! No sugar interventions or disruptions.

INSULIN SENSITIVITY AND RESISTANCE

Cells can become *insulin resistant* or decrease their insulin sensitivity when this sugar imbalance happens. Insulin resistance means that your cells no longer allow insulin to unlock them, so the insulin can't deposit the glucose. The insulin receptor on the cell can no longer be unlocked by the insulin. It's like all the cell "hotel rooms" changed their locks, so the insulin "hotel keeper" can't unlock them. This leads to a host of problems: for one, now the glucose has nowhere to go, so it stays in the blood, leading to a spike in blood sugar. Additionally, the cells can't get what they need because they don't have their energy source. This can lead to a craving for carbs. So, we have glucose running rampant and cells running on empty. No wonder this leads to so many problems!

The body's internal job is to maintain homeostasis, or balance. When the pancreas realizes that there's still glucose in the bloodstream, it kicks into high gear to produce even more insulin, to try to mediate the situation and try again to get the glucose into the cells. But since the cells are insulin resistant, it doesn't do any good.

Now the blood is swimming with extra glucose *and* insulin. Higher levels of insulin in the bloodstream make it more likely for you to gain weight, and higher levels of glucose lead to the symptoms of high blood sugar, or hyperglycemia: fatigue, trouble concentrating, headaches, and more. In addition, the pancreas can become damaged and overworked if it's continuing to make insulin that isn't helping.

QUICK CHECKLIST

You may have insulin resistance if:

- ❏ You frequently feel very, very hungry or very, very thirsty. This hunger can persist even after a meal, leading you to binge eat or to continue grazing all day long.
- ❏ You experience increased urination.
- ❏ You have tingling "pins and needles" sensations in your hands and feet.
- ❏ You suffer from fatigue and sleepiness, to the point that you're drinking cup after cup of coffee and still dragging through the day.

Your body's insulin sensitivity is simply how sensitive your cells are to insulin—in other words, whether they let insulin unlock their doors or not. The higher the sensitivity, the better. You can raise your insulin sensitivity with the anti-inflammatory lifestyle and environmental changes we will discuss in this book by mitigating stress on the body, getting more sleep, and eliminating the number of toxic stressors.

METABOLIC SYNDROME

Insulin resistance can lead to or be correlated with metabolic syndrome (also referred to as "syndrome X"), which means your body is experiencing three of the five risk factors that raise your risk for ischemic heart disease, diabetes, and stroke. The five risk factors are:

1. High blood pressure
2. High fasting blood sugar

3. Low HDL ("good") cholesterol level (higher levels of good cholesterol lessen the risk for stroke or heart attack)
4. High triglyceride level (fat found in the bloodstream)
5. A large waistline (or an "apple" shape due to fat around the waist, or obesity)

Aside from each of these risk factors, there are no real symptoms beyond gaining weight. So, many people actually have metabolic syndrome and don't know it. According to a 2018 report, it's estimated that one in three Americans has metabolic syndrome.[1] It isn't a disease like the name suggests, but rather it means that one in three Americans has at least three of the main risk factors for more serious implications, such as ischemic heart disease, diabetes, and stroke. Metabolic syndrome is becoming the "new normal"—and it shouldn't be. But, since more and more food chains, restaurants, and food manufacturers are loading foods up with sugar and cholesterol, the impacts have been significant.

QUICK CHECKLIST

You may have metabolic syndrome if:

❑ You notice that you have a growing waistline. As vague as that sounds, that's truly the only real noticeable "symptom" of metabolic syndrome!

❑ However, symptoms such as blurred vision, increased hunger or thirst, and fatigue can also be telltale signs that something is amiss.

Additionally, if you frequently look at nutritional labels, you may have noticed that "Sugars" falls under the "Total Carbohydrates" category. While the major nutritional information for the major players like protein, cholesterol, fat, and sodium is represented with their percentage of daily value (or their percentage of how much you should consume on a daily basis), sugar doesn't have a percentage. It only shows the percentage of total carbohydrates for the daily value.

This leads consumers to consume far more sugar than they should. A snack can boast that it's "fat-free" and therefore seems healthy but contains far more sugar than someone should consume on a daily basis. In fact, even snacks with labels such as "healthy," "organic," "natural," "gluten-free," or "vegan" can contain far more sugar than I would recommend you consume in an entire day! The less sugar, the better. When we look closer at how we've been taught to assess nutritional value in American consumerism, we see that sugar flies under the radar: a silent killer that wreaks havoc on our bodies, spiking our blood sugar and in general making us feel unwell.

That being said, "sugar-free" on a label doesn't mean it's healthy, either! It could be even worse: sugar-free, but still filled with chemicals and toxins that our body doesn't know how to identify. These toxins can lead to many horrible health complications. It's frustrating, I know. How are you supposed to know what's healthy to eat? Why can't you just trust that the foods you purchase are OK for you, and won't cause pain and other uncomfortable symptoms, and eventually lead to disease, even cancer?

Right now, you can't trust food labels or anything that's on the shelves in your grocery store, even if they appear to be "healthy." It's all part of a big marketing scheme that requires extra effort to identify which foods are truly healthy for you and are not just pretending to be; but with time and attention, you'll be able to easily notice which ones are labeled as "healthy" from a marketing ploy intended to get you hooked on their latest "healthy" snack.

It's not really your fault that you are consuming too much sugar (and I'm going to assume that you are, since according to Healthy Food America, 58% of Americans exceed the dietary guidelines).[2] It's not your fault—because food systems have lied to you in labeling and marketing and have dosed up your foods with unnecessary sugar since birth.

If you look at most of an infant's first foods, "sugar" is one of the main ingredients! It's actually disturbing. Why does a baby need sugar? Crackers, puffs, and pouches are often loaded with added syrups and sugars. Why does almost every salad dressing, cereal, condiment, frozen food, and packaged item have sugar added? Can't we just eat real food as it is?! We've never really had the chance.

Additionally, it's not your fault you're craving that sugar kick, because sugar is chemically addicting. Your brain gets a dopamine rush every time you indulge in something that's particularly sweet. When the crash occurs—the crash that sends you searching for caffeine, more sugar and carbs, or a nap—your body is actually craving *more sugar*. Even though you have already crashed your body with excessive amounts of sugar, and your "machine" gears have become sticky and hard to run, the body still craves more sugar . . . more of the very thing that's making it groggy and causing it to malfunction in the first place. Your body has become accustomed to the high blood sugar in your bloodstream, and when that abruptly stops, your blood sugar takes a dip—hence, the crash. The quickest (and most delicious) way to rebound from the crash is to take in more sugar. Thus the cycle continues. I'm sure you've experienced this . . . the day after eating a bunch of sugar, you crave carbs and sugar even more! You don't need sugar, but you crave it, so you continue to consume it. Big food and snack companies want this to happen, because that means you continue to purchase their sugar-filled food. You're addicted, which is great for their business and terrible for your health. Break the cycle. I challenge you. Grab a friend (you can pick me!) and let's ditch sugar together for good! I have the BEST swaps for all your sugary go-tos (even that wine you enjoy!). We can do this!

PREDIABETES AND TYPE 2 DIABETES

Over time, high levels of blood sugar can lead to the development of dangerous conditions, such as prediabetes. Prediabetes means that your blood sugar levels are higher than they should be, but they're not quite high enough to be diagnosed as type 2 diabetes per the written guidelines. That being said, for YOUR body in particular, even being prediabetic could be horribly damaging, and internally it can be just the same as being diabetic. Just because the laboratory tests don't quite define you as diabetic doesn't mean you don't have a serious problem to address within "the machine" in your body. If anything, being prediabetic should be a major wake-up call.

According to the CDC, 80% of you are walking around prediabetic, and you don't even know it![3] (Or you're diabetic for your individual body, as we are all biochemically unique and your "normal" sugar levels could run higher or lower than others' sugar levels.) It's also possible that you have developed diabetes, but you don't yet know it. In 2019, the International Diabetes Foundation published its ninth edition report that noted that *one in two adults with diabetes is undiagnosed.*[4]

In type 2 diabetes, the body doesn't respond to insulin in the way that it's supposed to, and insulin resistance occurs. Over time, an insulin deficiency also takes place because the pancreas simply can't produce any more. Blood sugar is higher than it should be, and the body can't handle the high amounts of glucose in the bloodstream.

> ## QUICK CHECKLIST
>
> *You may have prediabetes or type 2 diabetes if:*
>
> ❏ You are excessively hungry or thirsty, no matter how much you eat or drink.
> ❏ Sleep doesn't seem to help in the overbearing fatigue you experience.
> ❏ You're running to the restroom all the time to urinate.
> ❏ You're gaining weight. The pants are feeling a little snug lately.

HOW TO REGULATE YOUR SUGAR

If you suspect sugar inflammation or any of the above noted diagnoses, the best course of action is to make lifestyle changes that decrease the number of stressors on your body. (In this case, too much sugar is a stressor.) Some of the greatest risk factors for sugar inflammation leading to full-blown disease include lack of sleep, a sedentary lifestyle, and high blood pressure. Because I like to be a detective, my question for you would be: What is *causing* a lack of sleep and high blood pressure? Stress is a major cause of both. If we can get stress levels down, get longer hours of healthy sleep, and decrease blood pressure, the risks of prediabetes and insulin resistance may go down. Additionally, an active lifestyle can help with curbing stress and can generally help you to feel better. I don't mean that you need to become an avid crosstrainer or a marathon runner, but I don't want you to lead a sedentary lifestyle. Get outdoors and take a walk, go for a swim, play more with your kids. Just live a generally more active lifestyle, and you'll be on your way! Walking is such a great place to start—even something as simple as making a pact with yourself to park at the very back corner of the grocery store parking lot to get in a few more steps.

For more detailed advice on how to fight sugar inflammation, go to page 233.

6

PSYCHOLOGICAL STRESS

isa is the mom of two young children and wife to a husband in the medical field. She came to me because she was experiencing crippling anxiety—that constant, nervous twang and series of heart palpitations that made it difficult to sleep and uncomfortable to do just about anything. She had no idea where it was coming from, and despite her attempts to de-stress, it didn't seem to do much. Anxiety plagued her life.

According to the World Health Organization, one in three people worldwide suffers from some type of anxiety disorder.[1] Depression is considered to be the leading disability worldwide. These mental disorders and other symptoms of psychological stress—such as irritability, negative thoughts, worry, and excessive mental stress—can all be traced back to inflammation in the body, which, as we know, is the body's response to external stressors.

QUICK CHECKLIST

You may have psychological stress if:

❑ You feel anxiety, depression, irritability, worry, or abnormal fears.

Many believe that these major mental disorders are caused by a chemical imbalance, and while this can be true in some cases, I'm interested in the *cause* of the imbalance and the *cause* of the inflammation. When the body is inflamed and normal processes become disturbed, the brain's ability to make the proper neurotransmitters to keep the body's emotional and stress state in homeostasis is hindered. This can lead to depressive episodes, anxiety disorders, and general irritability and stress. Not to mention that many of these essential brain neurotransmitters are made in the gut lining, so a healthy gut and digestive system are needed for a healthy brain and mood.

Understanding psychological stress and mood disorders requires a holistic look at what's going on in each individual's life and all the stressors that are adding up to the Total Toxic Burden. In this case, psychological stress is significant! We live in an increasingly high-stress world that puts immense pressure on us to constantly be on our "A game" at work, to outdo ourselves, and to keep up with long work hours. We often wake up before the sun rises, we work all day with little rest, and we finally make it to bed long after the sun sets.

In addition to busy schedules, there can be situational stress that arises in our lives. Stress from problems at work, stress from family dynamics, stress from big life changes such as moving homes or moving cities . . . you could even potentially be stressed about a vacation that's coming up, even if you're excited about the vacation and it's a "good thing." Excitement can be misinterpreted as stress, especially if it takes up a lot of mental real estate. Imagine that you're leaving for a European tour in a few weeks, so you lie awake at night mentally making a planning list, making sure you're making progress on your to-do lists for train tickets, rental cars, and hotel reservations, and feeling anxious for the long flight.

"Did I remember to pack socks? Do I even need socks? Will that extra pair of shoes fit in my carry-on? I hope my charging adaptors work. What if . . . [fill in the blank with whatever your mind is brewing up to worry about!]?"

This can be perceived by your body as stress, and it can cause inflammation.

Knowing that you're going through a time when you're more susceptible to stress is important so that you can be extra cognizant of the total stressors affecting you and how they're stacking up to your Total Toxic Burden. I'm also concerned with chronic stress: that constant sense of worry or overwhelmed feeling that can operate under the surface, causing inflammation even if you don't know it. Over time, this leads to the imbalance of the body and inflammation, and can cause even *more* stress, as well as symptoms of anxiety and depression. Remember, right now we are focused solely on psychological stress, but stress from your environment and food can place just as much, if not more, harm on your body.

NEUROTRANSMITTERS

First, let's understand what regulates our mood and feelings to begin with. The brain and nerve cells produce and fire chemical messengers called "neurotransmitters," which act as the built-in mailman for the body. The brain has a message to send? The neurotransmitters are on it! Their "mail route" is throughout the nervous system, and they're fired the moment the brain has a message to send. They bring those messages, like letters, to different cells, notifying them to perform different functions such as digestion, heart rate, sleep cycles, appetite, and—most importantly for this chapter—mood. They do it so well that they give the United States postal system a run for its money!

There are over one hundred neurotransmitters in the body that scientists have discovered to date, and each has one of three functions. The first is an excitatory neurotransmitter, which, true to its name, "excites" or encourages a cell to take action. Then, an inhibitory neurotransmitter inhibits or discourages a cell from taking action. Finally, modulatory transmitters are able to send messages to many neurons at the same time, as well as communicate with other neurotransmitters.

Some of the most well-known neurotransmitters include dopamine, which we think of as the "pleasure" neurotransmitter. When you do something that brings you pleasure (like a super relaxing, alone-time spa day with a massage, my personal favorite!) or eat something divine that you may look forward to (like organic dark chocolate–dipped strawberries), dopamine is released.

Then, endorphins send an energizing, feel-good wave throughout the body. This is also the reason for the feel-good "high" you may get after a great workout, because endorphins can also be produced after exercise. If you've ever run long distances, you may be familiar with the jolt of energy and good feelings you get once you're recovering after exercise. Endorphins also work as pain relievers.

Then there's serotonin, the "happy hormone." This is another neurotransmitter that regulates mood and helps us to feel happier and more energized. Exposure to natural sunlight is one of the ways our body produces serotonin, which is why research cited in *Brain: A Journal of Neurology* has found that seasonal affective disorder (SAD)—when lower moods are experienced in the dark of winter or in cloud-covered cities like Seattle—is linked to a decrease in serotonin.[2] So, next time you're feeling a bit down or sleepy, get outside and feel the sun on your skin. Bring a good book (maybe head out there with this one right this second!), listen to an inspirational podcast, or just take time in nature to be silent—it helps.

These neurotransmitters create a dance with other neurotransmitters and other hormones, and levels among one type of neurotransmitter or hormone can influence levels among others. They all influence one another, rather than working separately. After all, they're a team. For example, an increase in serotonin from a fun day at the beach can lead to a decrease in cortisol levels, which is the hormone associated with stress. Wins! As with most processes in the body, this neuro dance of different hormones and neurotransmitters requires a perfect balance. When under constant stress, or when there is other inflammation in the body, the brain—which is connected to every part of the body—is impacted.

There's a popular assumption that, when we're under great stress or experiencing psychological disorders such as depression or anxiety, it's the result of a specific chemical imbalance within the brain, such as the malproduction of our feel-good neurotransmitters: serotonin and dopamine. And many are made to believe that this "chemical imbalance" is just the way that they were born, and the cards that they were dealt. It's true that these are real chemical imbalances, but I've found that we can actually rewire and rebalance these levels to get you feeling amazing, just as you should! In fact, recent literature states that a chemical imbalance isn't actually always to blame for depression and anxiety; it can be other factors as well.

Actually, just believing that a chemical imbalance you're "stuck with" causes depression could lead to further depressed and negative feelings. Researchers from the University of Wyoming conducted a study to determine the effects of believing that one's depressive episodes are caused by a chemical imbalance.[3] They conducted their study with two groups of people who had been diagnosed with depression, giving each a "Rapid Depression Test," in which they swabbed the inside of each participant's cheek, then ran a test on the saliva sample. The control group was told that there actually was not a chemical imbalance (low levels of serotonin) in their test result. The test group was shown a graph depicting their very low levels of serotonin in their brains—in other words, they were told and shown that they had a chemical imbalance.

After seeing the results, each participant completed a measures packet with questions about their depressive episodes and their beliefs regarding the causes of each. The researchers found something interesting when reviewing the results of the test group's packets. By telling the test participants that their depressive episodes were the result of a chemical imbalance, they had "activated a host of negative beliefs with the potential to worsen the course of depression." The study also went on to find that this chemical imbalance feedback "lowered individuals' perceived ability to successfully regulate their depressed moods, particularly via cognitive mood."

Now, this doesn't mean that there's no markable cause within every brain scan of someone experiencing anxiety, depression, negative thoughts, or a down mood. Scientists simply haven't been able to find significant research with trends in one way or another. You'd expect that people with depression symptoms would have low levels of serotonin in the brain, but there are also many people who have been diagnosed with depression who actually are producing enough serotonin. One thing's for sure: something is off within the body and the brain that causes these symptoms, but it's not always what we think it is.

Rather than pointing blindly to a chemical imbalance, recent research has instead found a link between inflammation and depression, anxiety, and other mood disorders.[4][5] Surprise!

Inflammation is to blame once again, and it causes an imbalance within the body that impacts emotions and moods, causing the mental disorders that can have a seriously detrimental impact on our lives. By understanding how inflammation has an effect on psychological stress, we can work to decrease inflammatory stressors so the body can heal. The link between the brain and every part of the body is significant, so it's no wonder that the brain's functionality can be hijacked, too, when inflammation and the immune system are waging an internal war.

DEPRESSION

Depression is described not only as the sense of feeling "down" or "sad" but more generally as the lack of feeling anything. This "numbness" or sense of emptiness can lead to a lack of interest in doing the things you typically love to do. It can interfere with sleep—either making sleep difficult or causing you to sleep too much—make it difficult to remember things or make decisions, reduce appetite or induce cravings, and create irritability and angry outbursts.

When someone is diagnosed with depression, psychiatrists typically prescribe antidepressants to help, which are intended to balance the brain's neurotransmitters to lead to an increase in appetite, energy, and mood. However, it's estimated that 10–30% of patients with depression do not see significant improvements from taking antidepressants.[6] Antidepressants act as a Band-Aid to the real problem—especially if a chemical imbalance isn't actually to blame for the symptoms. Worse, many antidepressants can cause side effects such as nausea, blurred vision, increased appetite, weight gain, insomnia, or fatigue. Now, there are times (for sure!) when pharmaceutical medications are needed. I just don't want you to feel that it's your only option or your lifelong option, as we've seen tremendous results in clients who were previously suffering from anxiety, depression, and other psychological imbalances thrive through lifestyle and anti-inflammatory changes.

QUICK CHECKLIST

You may be experiencing depression if:

❏ You feel sad or numb far more often than you feel happy.

❏ The sadness is tinged with irritability, feelings of guilt, or hopelessness; and the activities that used to make you happy do little to help.

❏ You are overwhelmingly fatigued, so much so that it seems like too much to get out of bed.

❏ You have many restless nights and can't get a full night's sleep.

❏ You are either excessively hungry or don't have an appetite at all.

In search of new solutions, researchers have continued to study depression, its causes, and the potential treatment options and, in doing so, have found a link between inflammation and depressive symptoms. Research from Emory University's School of Medicine stated that "chronic exposure to increased inflammation is thought to drive changes in neurotransmitters . . . that lead to depressive symptoms and that may also interfere with or circumvent the efficacy of antidepressants." It also notes that numerous studies have found elevated inflammatory cytokines in people with depression.[7]

In light of these repeatable results, scientists have started to explore behavioral immunology, or the link between the brain and the immune system. In fact, Emory University has devoted a department to the study, and it's currently studying the link between depression and immunology at the time this book is written.

ANXIETY

Closely linked to depression is anxiety. Think back to a time when you were nervous for a big work or school presentation. Maybe you could hear your heartbeat in your ears, your knees were shaking, and it was hard to get a full breath. Or, maybe something is going on in the world (or your world!) that makes you nervous about the unknown, and you have this pit, this anxious feeling in your body that's hard to explain, but is definitely not your "normal." Or, maybe you're feeling irritable and stressed without any real reason as to why.

When anxiety is present, stress hormones go haywire, and this causes not just the anxiety and nervousness but also other harmful changes within the body due to elevated stress levels and an activated sympathetic nervous state, which is the running-from-a-bear fight-or-flight state.

So many experience this inflammation from anxiety on a daily basis—even just while sitting at work or driving to meet friends at brunch. Even while trying to choose a nail polish color for a pedicure at the salon, the anxiety of indecision can creep in! These types of situations should not cause so much anxiety and distress in our body, and it's something we really need to focus inward about. We need to—and can!—alter our mindset to a more balanced and calming state.

QUICK CHECKLIST

You may suffer from anxiety if:

❑ You frequently feel nervous or anxious.

❏ You experience heart palpitations, where your heart beats irregularly, skips a beat, or beats too quickly.

❏ You experience nausea, diarrhea, and/or insomnia as a result of the anxiety.

❏ Your thoughts are racing and it's difficult to concentrate.

This is what anxiety feels like. Those with anxiety know that there's no real reason to feel anxious necessarily, but they feel it anyway. And they feel it constantly. Or, the anxiety can show up as excessive worry about something in a person's life, as an attempt to "validate" the feeling, which only leads to more of it! Imagine that your daughter is at her best friend's house for a sleepover, where she's slept over dozens of times before. Anxiety could present itself as the constant need to check in on her, to make sure she's OK, to call the best friend's parents . . . even if you just checked in thirty minutes ago and they were having the time of their lives. Logically, you know that everything is OK, but the excessive worry persists.

For my client Lisa, the anxiety had become chronic—and she's not the only client (or friend!) I've worked with who has experienced constant feelings of stress and nervousness. We all feel anxious from time to time, and for some of us, it's more constant. It can lead to symptoms beyond the "I'm nervous!" feeling, such as heart palpitations, trouble sleeping, irritability, restlessness, and gastrointestinal problems from the stress. One of the most frustrating aspects of anxiety is how it seems to spring forth without any reason. When we're nervous to get onstage or take an important phone call, we can sometimes talk ourselves out of the nerves, or at least expect that we'll feel a cool wave of relief when it's finally over. The sense that we don't know where the anxiety comes from can make us feel powerless. That's why it can be empowering to understand that inflammation is causing it—which means there are stressors in your environment, diet, and life that are causing it. Once we fix those, the body can return to homeostasis and you can feel like yourself again more often. You may still feel "anxious" at times, but a normal type of anxiousness, not a debilitating one.

In addition to studies on the role of inflammation in influencing depression, there is a line of research that suggests inflammation can influence anxiety, too. Anxiety and depression are commonly experienced together—according to Beth Salcedo, MD, 60% of people with anxiety will also experience the symptoms of depression.[8] It's not clear why this is, but a 2010 study from the University of Western Ontario identified a biological link between stress, depression, and anxiety, and the research specifically noted that "the causes for both (anxiety and depression) are strongly linked to stressful experiences."[9]

We know that stress causes the body to become inflamed, and that inflammation can lead to both anxiety and depression. Anxiety, particularly, causes even more stress in the body, which creates a circuit of repetition that leaves the body chronically inflamed and chronically anxious. The only way to stop the cycle of anxiety is to address the inflammation . . . by addressing the stress. This is why practices such as meditation and yoga are frequently advised for people with anxiety—but there are many other healthy ways to cope with stress as well. It's about what works best for you and restores your peace.

Maybe "burning off" the extra energy by running a few miles every day and working up a sweat will work best. Maybe taking time to find your center and get control of your breath in a hot yoga class will work best. You owe it to yourself to continue finding new ways to mitigate what's overwhelming you, be it making changes to your work-life schedule, meeting weekly with a therapist or psychologist, or even speaking more regularly with a trusted friend. This stress mitigation leads to inflammation mitigation, which can lessen the symptoms of anxiety and depression. It's too important to ignore! Self-care truly has implications far beyond just taking a few relaxing hours off from work and errands.

For more nutritional and exercise tips tailored to you, go to page 233.

EXCESSIVE MENTAL STRESS

Not only can stress cause inflammation that influences anxiety and depression, but inflammation can also cause even *more stress* in and of itself. You read that right: however you frame it, there's usually a link between psychological stress and inflammation. While it certainly makes sense that the body becomes inflamed to prepare for a fight-or-flight response when you're feeling stressed, even more interesting is how inflammation can also cause *more* feelings of stress because of its influence on anxiety and depression. It's an endless cycle.

Sheldon Cohen, a professor of psychology from Carnegie Mellon University, found that unregulated inflammation arises from stress when there's a problem with cortisol sensitivity.[10] For background, cortisol is your body's built-in stress response system. If you're pulling through an intersection and another car doesn't see you and almost hits you, the moment of panic causes the release of cortisol. You may even be able to recollect this feeling in your body! You become flushed, your heart starts to race, and your breathing becomes ragged. According to Cohen, "prolonged stress alters the effectiveness of cortisol to regulate the inflammatory response because it decreases tissue sensitivity to the hormone." The more stress that's felt, the more inflammation occurs—which leads to numerous other symptoms.

Stress creates the continuation of a war within the body. The longer the body is under stress, the less the body is able to heal and fulfill its normal functioning processes of handling stress, handling inflammation, and regulating the balanced production of hormones and neurotransmitters to stabilize mood, emotions, and other functionalities. What a mess!

QUICK CHECKLIST

You may have excessive mental stress if:

- ❏ You are overwhelmingly fatigued and slow-moving.
- ❏ You are anxious and worry incessantly.
- ❏ The anxiety is paired with a racing heart, which can cause chest pains.
- ❏ You commonly get headaches and feel pain throughout your body via aches and tight muscles.
- ❏ You frequently come down with colds or other infections; your immune system seems to be low.

CONNECTION BETWEEN THE GUT AND THE BRAIN

What many don't know is that there's also a connection between the gut and the brain that can contribute to symptoms of anxiety and depression. The gut is sometimes even referred to as your "second brain," because it's essentially the brain's sidekick or its "mini-me"! The gut has the enteric nervous system (ENS), which is composed of one hundred million nerve cells within the lining of the digestive tract. Each of these nerve cells communicates with the brain, and vice versa, so there's a direct line between the two. Talk about efficiency.

Dr. Jay Pasricha, director of the Johns Hopkins Center for Neurogastroenterology, noted that "for decades, researchers and doctors thought that anxiety and depression contributed to these problems. But our studies and others show that it may also be the other way around."[11] Gut problems can contribute to both depression and anxiety. "These new findings may explain why a higher-than-normal percentage of people with IBS and functional bowel problems develop depression and anxiety," Pasricha added.

If the microbiota composition of the gut is off, the brain will feel the impact. We'll unpack more about this in the next chapter on digestive inflammation, but when the digestive system is irritated and inflamed, it's unable to function properly—leading to an inability to absorb the proper nutrients from the food that you consume. Those nutrients are needed for the brain to produce the "feel-good" neurotransmitters that keep us happy, calm, and balanced, such as serotonin and dopamine.

When Lisa came to me because of her anxiety, we got to work evaluating her stressors holistically. Specifically, we pinpointed the cause in her diet and digestive system. She had been experiencing some digestive distress, which led to psychological distress through the enteric nervous system. This had also become cyclical, because feeling anxious can lead to even more digestive distress.

Once we changed her diet and addressed some of the bad bacteria that were causing issues in her digestive lining, you'll never believe what happened. She emailed me after just one week of beginning the changes, over the moon because her anxiety had decreased by about 75 percent. Wow! Major changes— and as thrilled as I am when a client's life changes quickly, it never surprises me anymore, because it's always traced back to inflammation and its root causes When we look beyond what's "wrong" with the person—the diagnosis, the symptoms, and the pains—and instead look to their environment and inflammatory inputs, we can make so many positive changes in the mind and environment that the body is able to heal itself. Although Lisa's symptoms decreased by 75 percent in ONE week, we didn't stop there. It takes a while for the body to fully rebalance and maintain long-term health, which is what I'm after.

So, to summarize: the imbalance of the gut leads to the imbalance of the brain and its neurotransmitters, and vice versa. And, since psychological stress can contribute to both uncomfortable GI symptoms *and* mental complications like depression and anxiety, it is all interconnected. The way to mediate it? Addressing the causes of inflammation within your life and implementing changes to rebalance it inside and out.

RESOLVING PSYCHOLOGICAL STRESS

There are a number of ways to reduce stress, and it's mainly about finding what works for you. Just as the peak of my health problems came when I was stressed about my postgrad decisions, many of my clients experience a correlation between their mental stress and the painful, uncomfortable, and distracting symptoms of inflammation throughout their body.

Notice that stress usually brings your body beyond its Total Toxic Burden. So, when going through a stressful time—or if you anticipate that one is coming up because of a work schedule or otherwise—take time to really check in with yourself and make sure all your other stressors are reduced or eliminated. This means following the tips I'll share in this book, and not just related to your mindfulness and mindset. It's also about things like replacing air filtration systems in your home, using water filters, eating nutritious and healthy anti-inflammatory foods, and dealing with stress in a healthy way: exercise, meditation, breath work, therapy, you name it!

The longer that your body is in a place of excessive stress, the more damage will be done. Inflammation in one area of your body can spread to, or influence, the inflammatory response in another area of your body. Symptoms can diversify, expand, and intensify as a result. Your mind is powerful, and while stress happens frequently in our lives, finding ways to cope with stress is an important step that will serve you for the rest of your life.

For more detailed nutrition and lifestyle tips tailored for you, go to page 233.

7

DIGESTIVE INFLAMMATION

A client of mine, Marcy, is a high-powered entrepreneur and CEO with a busy work and travel schedule. She was always jet-setting off to new cities for conferences, meetings, and events. And she was hosting her own events as well, multiple times a year, speaking and having to be fully "on" for days in a row, from a.m. to p.m.

Her job was "fun," and she loved what she did, but man was it tiring. The late nights and the constant brain power started to take a toll on her. Managing a team, implementing ideas, and making deadlines started to break down her energy.

On the outside, she was a powerful, vibrant, fit, energetic go-getter and businesswoman, but on the inside her body was at war—and she felt it.

Marcy tried to avoid the inflammation however she could. She pushed back the symptoms of anxiety, fatigue, bloating, constipation. She covered them up with every pill, powder, or "hack" so she could keep moving faster and just "get through."

Thinking her symptoms could be a result of her diet, she would spend a great deal of time and care packing healthy lunches to take to work and on work trips so she could nix eating conference food, and bringing healthy snacks along for plane rides, but it didn't seem to help. Other people thought she was so dedicated and awesome for eating "healthy" all the time, but to her it was a frustrating battle of trying to do "all the right things" and still having problems. Her digestive inflammation showed up as bloating: rock-hard bloating that was painful to the touch and happened almost every single time she ate anything—even healthy salads. Sometimes it was so severe that she couldn't fit into any of the clothing she had packed for her trip and needed to go out last minute to buy something baggier to cover up her bloating and hide the "evidence" of her health battles or not-so-great late-night meal option. The discomfort led to her missing many important meetings and client dinners because she was embarrassed and simply didn't feel well, which only led to more stress. She was frustrated, especially because she was being hyper cognizant of what she was eating. She was tired of faking smiles and coming up with excuses as to why she was so sorry, but she once again couldn't make that social hour, dinner party, morning meeting, and so forth. She got through what she needed to, then just wanted to hide away in her room, get into baggy clothes, get under her covers, and hold her belly, ashamed and annoyed.

When she came to me, she had reached her wit's end. She started her phone conversation with confidence and energy, just as she always portrayed, but after a few questions from me about how she was really feeling, her voice became shaky and quiet, and I knew there were tears forming on the other line. "Marcy?" I asked.

She gathered herself to respond. "What do I do, Maggie? . . . I need help."

Finally—her tough external shell was softening up to let me in. She finally was ready to accept help and put her health into someone else's hands, mine, so she could focus on what she does best—running her business—while I focused on what I do best—helping high-performing women get their health back.

Marcy was really trying to do "everything right": eating organic and gluten-free foods, prioritizing fitness, journaling each morning . . . the works. And yet she felt miserable inside and knew it. Her digestive issues weren't the only issues. . . . Now they were coupled with weight gain, disturbed sleep, and an onset of anxiety and even depressive feelings. Her motivation was lacking—so unlike her. Her drive was slipping away.

Marcy wasn't the first client who came to me with digestive issues, and she won't be the last, either. When your constipation, bloating, and/or diarrhea begin to interfere with your life, your work, and your happiness, it's time to make a change. It's time to look at the stressors that may be causing digestive inflammation in your life and fix them for good.

QUICK CHECKLIST

You may have digestive inflammation if:

- ❏ You can't remember the last time you weren't bloated.
- ❏ People out there actually have normal and regular bowel movements?!
- ❏ You sometimes have to run to the bathroom, ASAP.
- ❏ You sometimes can't remember the last time you had a bowel movement because it's been so long.
- ❏ You have pain in your abdomen, so bad that it hurts to eat and hurts even more to have a bowel movement.

❏ You're either battling with weight loss or weight gain, and they're equally horrible.

❏ Your energy is in the tank—sometimes you feel like your ninety-seven-year-old grandma has more energy than you do.

❏ You're dizzy, exhausted, and unmotivated.

UNDERSTANDING THE DIGESTIVE SYSTEM AND INFLAMMATION

To understand the digestive system, let's first go through a quick overview of what happens when the body digests something. After food has been chewed, it takes a ride down the esophagus and into the stomach, where gastric acid breaks it down further and kills bacteria. Then it moves into the small intestine, where most of the nutrient absorption is done. Nutrients are absorbed via the "villi," which are in the small intestine's ridges, as the digested food passes through.

Its next route is through the large intestine, which is responsible for reabsorbing any extra water and bile to make the stool solid. This entire process is run by your autonomic nervous system, so of course you don't have to consciously think about any of it in order for it to function properly.

Or . . . do you? If you're always in a sympathetic and stressed state, your digestive system will consequently perform poorly, and won't break down your food fully or properly absorb the nutrients you're eating. So, in Marcy's case, it wasn't exactly WHAT she was eating, it was HOW her body was able to absorb and use those nutrients. Her body was under constant stress. She loved her job and thrived in the high-stress, high-demanding atmosphere. She loved the competition and grit it took to climb to the top and consistently raise her own bar.

However, that stress, even when it was for something really exciting, needed to find a balance that would allow her internal body to thrive.

What you eat and the toxins you expose yourself to are also very, very important. Inflammation can happen within the intestines as a result of ingested offenders such as pathogens or irritants, and persistent inflammatory stimuli can lead to chronic inflammation.[1] As we'll learn, irritants such as parasites and heavy metals can disturb the microbiota of the gut. When inflammation occurs as a result of these bacterial intruders, things don't work the way they should—leading to conditions such as irritable bowel syndrome (IBS), nutrient malabsorption, food intolerance, and unpleasant symptoms such as diarrhea and constipation.

It's OK to not be OK right now. It's not OK to not do anything about it. You don't have to accept this as who you are or your new story. Your past and your current state do not have to be your future. YOU decide from here.

IRRITABLE BOWEL SYNDROME (IBS)

One of the most common issues that can occur in the digestive system is irritable bowel syndrome, or IBS. Between 10–25% of the world's population has this syndrome.[2]

However, the truth is that IBS is simply a term used to identify symptoms that are happening within someone's digestion. It's not a "real answer" to anything, and it is in no way a root cause of your symptoms. The true root cause of your symptoms can likely be taken care of and balanced with the strategies you'll find in this book.

Remember, the large intestine's job is to reabsorb liquid from the stool, and it needs to do this on a precise timeline in order for it to not be too liquid or too solid. With IBS, either the large intestine contracts too quickly, hurrying the stool along before enough water has been absorbed, which results in diarrhea. Or it can contract too slowly, which means too much water reabsorption happens and the stool becomes too hard. This causes constipation. Many who have IBS experience a ping-ponging between the two: a phase with constipation, then a phase with diarrhea, and back and forth.

Symptoms of IBS include abdominal pain for at least three days out of the month, with a connection between the pain and bathroom use, and change in stool form (very liquid or very solid). Essentially, as long as a clear correlation or causation can be established between the abdominal pain and the stool, it's likely that your doctor will term this as irritable bowel syndrome.

QUICK CHECKLIST

You may have IBS if:

- ❏ You commonly experience both diarrhea and constipation, usually alternating.
- ❏ You have mood challenges, such as depression and anxiety.
- ❏ You have pain in your abdomen, and it hurts worse right before a bowel movement.
- ❏ You can't figure out what's going on with your body. Sometimes you feel "fine" and other times you're absolutely miserable (but really, you never feel AMAZING now that you think of it. It's a

baseline of "blah" and just getting through most days).

❑ You wish you could go just one day without feeling inflamed and in pain.

❑ You wish you could eat just one burger and have a beer without waking up the next day paying for it big-time.

❑ You have horrible symptoms, even when you eat perfectly.

❑ You just wish your stomach was normal again.

❑ Working is really hard, because you never know when you're going to need to run to the bathroom.

POOR DIGESTION OR ABSORPTION OF NUTRIENTS

Now, remember that the digestive system's chief responsibility is to absorb the nutrients through what you eat (then discard what you don't need). The entire reason we eat is to get nutrients and energy! My grandma always said, "Eat to live, don't live to eat." She's super fit and healthy even in her older age and looks so incredibly young. She's never had a weight issue in her life and appears to be bursting with more energy than most people would know what to do with. She's basically super grandma.

Fun personal fact: I'm named after her!

I now eat in a way that, for the most part, allows me to feel amazing. Why? Because I'm obsessed with feeling on top of the world! I can't stand it if I feel groggy, drained, bloated, or swollen. I want to feel energetic and healthy every single day. I want to look in the mirror and see a strong and vibrant "me." I eat well and consciously choose nutrient-dense and whole, real foods instead of packaged foods because it makes me feel this way. So that's what I prioritize.

QUICK CHECKLIST

You may have malabsorption if:

❏ You experience stomach cramping, bloating, or distension.
❏ You commonly have diarrhea and/or gas.
❏ Your stool appears pale or white.
❏ You feel very weak and fatigued.

When I eat a varied and diverse diet that is full of colorful vegetables of all different kinds, it sounds silly but I can actually feel the nutrients going through my body. It's true! I think about it and can envision it happening. When I drink that homemade smoothie with the ingredients I have carefully chosen so that I can give my mind and my body the best start to the day and the most energy possible, I can visualize the goodness going through every cell, every organ, every vein. I'm addicted to feeling great, and eating for nutrients is one way I do this.

So, the small intestine's functionality is quite important for our health. This is what gets you the fats, carbohydrates, proteins, vitamins, and electrolytes from the food you consume. It's what makes sure we feel GOOD from all the foods we're eating! If something becomes off-balanced in the digestive system, a number of uncomfortable symptoms can happen, such as bloating, diarrhea, constipation, fatigue, stomach cramping, abdominal pain, and a general feeling of weakness.

Specifically, when the small intestine isn't working properly and absorbing nutrients, it's referred to as "malabsorption." This means that the digestive system is malfunctioning in its role of absorbing nutrients from what you consume during the digestive process. You could be eating super healthy, but it doesn't matter if you have malabsorption—you'll still be nutrient deficient, which is a big problem. This can result in weakness, hair loss, fatigue, weight gain, or weight loss, and it also may appear as the sudden need to run to the restroom after you eat. The symptoms may differ depending on which specific nutrients are not being absorbed correctly. For example, edema (fluid retention in the body) can happen from protein malabsorption; muscle cramping can occur from the malabsorption of vitamin D, calcium, and potassium; and anemia (marked by feeling exhausted and weak) can occur from the malabsorption of iron, folic acid, and vitamin B12.

This chronic malabsorption is often referred to as "malabsorption syndrome." There are a number of reasons why this can be caused, but inflammation of the intestines is one of the most common, or inflammation from other diseases in the gallbladder, liver, and pancreas that can contribute to malabsorption. Bad bacteria or a parasite can damage the gut lining in the small intestine, which makes it challenging for nutrients to be absorbed. When the intestine walls become inflamed because of an imbalance in the digestive system, it becomes more challenging for the small intestine to absorb nutrients in the way it's supposed to. In this case, you could be eating the healthiest foods in the world—leafy green smoothies, lean proteins—and your body would not absorb any of the nutrients.

This can also be caused by heightened stress, and by eating habits such as eating quickly, always eating on the go, or yo-yo dieting, which means you restrict what you eat sometimes, then binge on certain foods and overeat at other times. Even if the foods you're bingeing on are healthy, these eating patterns are still damaging.

Malabsorption can also have an effect on the brain, resulting in anxiety, depression, and other markers of psychological distress. If the body can't adequately absorb nutrients, the brain doesn't create the hormones it needs to regulate the body's emotional state. Gut inflammation can be the first domino in a series, leading to more symptoms, complications, and a general sense of dis-ease.

FOOD INTOLERANCE

Sometimes clients come to me because they suddenly developed symptoms around a food that they had previously eaten for all their life with no problem. They wonder if they have suddenly developed a late-onset allergy to the food. A true allergic reaction happens within the immune system and can be life-threatening, and it is usually experienced through hives, rash, difficulty breathing, nausea, stomach pain, swelling, and shortness of breath. Most of the time, when you're experiencing nagging symptoms that aren't immediately life-threatening but are definitely frustrating, it's likely food intolerance or sensitivity. Instead of a full-blown allergic reaction to the food, a food intolerance results in more chronic nagging symptoms, such as headache or migraine, anxiety and irritability, bloating and constipation or diarrhea, weight gain, skin rashes, swelling, dizziness, or pain.

QUICK CHECKLIST

You may have a food intolerance if you experience:
- ❏ Nausea, vomiting, or diarrhea
- ❏ Gas, stomach pains, and cramping
- ❏ Heartburn
- ❏ Nervousness or anxiety
- ❏ Headaches
- ❏ Aches and pains

❑ Weight gain
❑ Skin rashes
❑ Acne
❑ Constipation
❑ Depression
❑ Insomnia
❑ Fatigue
❑ Autoimmune disease

It's definitely a good idea to visit an allergist if there's confusion about whether you have an allergy or a food intolerance, but a good rule of thumb is that the symptoms of a food intolerance take a bit longer to appear than those of an allergic reaction. For example: if you eat a crab leg and you're allergic to crab, it will only be a few minutes before you start to experience the scary and uncomfortable symptoms of an allergic reaction: swelling of the throat, difficulty breathing, hives, or other markers of allergies. But if you eat that crab leg and you're intolerant or sensitive to crab, you may feel more irritable, swollen, or in pain. You may have trouble sleeping that night or gain a few pounds that week. The symptoms are less immediately severe, but definitely still present.

An allergist will be able to do an allergy test to determine if you have any true "allergies." If that test comes back negative, or nonsignificant to you (meaning you are allergic to certain random foods, but you never consume them so it wouldn't explain your symptoms), then definitely seek out a functional medicine practitioner to complete a blood-draw test to determine your specific food intolerances and what to do about them. In my business, this is something we do often for our clientele.

Food intolerances can develop for a number of reasons. It could be digestion-related, when the digestion slows down and the body stops or slows the release of the enzymes needed to break down certain foods. This can happen as a result of inflammation or an imbalance within the digestive system that prevents the normal release of the enzymes you need. Or it can happen as a result of the specific foods you're consuming, because they may be inherently inflammatory and push your body's capacity beyond its Total Toxic Burden whenever you eat them.

Food intolerance can also develop from eating the same things day in and day out. Are you the type of person who follows the exact same grocery list at the grocery store each week? Could you recite your daily breakfast, lunch, and dinner to me that you've had consistently for weeks on end, without much diversity at all? It's likely that you will develop a food intolerance by eating this way. Not to mention, you'll deplete your body of essential nutrients from the varied and diverse foods it needs to properly populate your gut lining, strengthen the immune system, decrease inflammation, and overall, to function at its best.

Another cause of food intolerance could be your eating habits—or, how and when you eat. If you eat under stress, rushing through each bite, scarfing down your meal so you can get on with your next task . . . or even if you eat aimlessly while simultaneously working at your desk, your body will not be able to properly break down and digest your food. This can lead to a possible food intolerance. So, mindful eating and your specific habits around *how* you eat really do matter a great deal.

Many practitioners don't ever ask about, consider, or assess if you have a food intolerance. In fact, most practitioners don't even ask for details about your nutrition at all—it's bizarre. I mean, you're here telling them you're suffering horribly with the most annoying symptoms, and they don't even bother to ask you about what you're putting in your mouth every day, your stress, sleep, lifestyle, if a recent trauma occurred—nothing! They simply give you that pill to help that symptom and send you on your way. The ones who do address food intolerance may "treat it" by telling you to nix gluten, dairy, corn, or other "common" food intolerances from your diet for a period of time. While it's true that there are certain foods that cause complications in a majority of individuals, it's not a one-size-fits-all fix if you actually want to get well long-term. AND you can't just take the food out and magically heal. You do need to still address the root cause and rebalance the damage done. Many of my clients have followed some sort of "elimination diet" or other removal of "top offending foods" to a T, but they become frustrated when their symptoms still don't resolve—like Marcy, who was following elimination diets yet still had symptoms. The reason you may be doing "everything right" and still feel sick, groggy, and bloated may be because you have a food intolerance to a food that's technically "allowed" on the prescribed elimination diet—even to something that's viewed as healthy, like apples, avocados, spinach, or celery.

Clients of mine have had food intolerances to anything from black pepper to romaine lettuce. It can be as random as it sounds. You won't know *for sure* what your food intolerance is until you have specialty functional medicine laboratory testing done—and it's advised to do so eventually, because elimination diets don't always solve the problem.

Another problem I have with these "diets" is that simply removing a specific food from your diet is not going to solve the problem—period. It likely wasn't the romaine lettuce, lemon, or whatever intolerance you have that caused your body to begin to experience symptoms. Those things developed AFTER the years of mental stress and poor lifestyle habits. It was the toxic-ities that enter your body from your home, hygiene products, or processed food choices. It was the way you ate, the long-term dieting, the binge eating, the fast foods. You must address and heal the true root cause of the intolerances if you want to heal your body, and to do so requires more than simply eliminating a handful of "bad foods" from your diet—whether you found a list online or a practitioner gave it to you. Taking out some foods is definitely helpful, but it's not the final answer. Allowing your internal body to completely rewire, heal, rebalance takes time. There's not a switch inside you that, after twenty-one days of taking out gluten and dairy, can switch everything in your "machine" back to normal and allow it to run again, better than ever. Nope. You may feel a little better, a few of the "gears" inside of your machine may turn a little faster, but eventually you'll break down again. Instead, you must allow the body adequate time to remove the offenders and replenish nutritional status by rewiring both your mindset and your daily lifestyle choices. Then, and only then, can you truly live fully again—free of stress and toxicities holding you back. So yes, we need to remove some foods for a time, but it's really about knowing how foods react inside and hurt your body, and how other foods heal it, then consciously choosing the ones that heal. It's also about repairing the damage that has already been done.

Your food can heal you, or it can break you.

Now, as I've said, testing is the gold standard for determining what food intolerances you may have. Get tested if you and your practitioner feel strongly that it's the right route for you. But I also want you to know that even without any laboratory testing at all, you can start to reduce your digestive inflammation right now if you follow the anti-inflammation tips presented in this book— down to your diet, environment, and eliminating stressors. By adhering to the advice in this guide, you are likely to notice some phenomenal and maybe even miraculous improvements in your health. I've had clients send me photos of their skin clearing up, their face changing shape, their decreasing weight, their abdomen going from looking six months pregnant to being flat. I've also had clients report that they're sleeping better than ever, their anxiety is nearly gone, and they have never been so focused because the brain fog has lifted. All these symptoms cleared from some simple food swaps! You will see all these results— improvements in mood, energy, sleep, weight, and more—by implementing changes in the gut because the body is rebalancing and strengthening head to toe when we feed it correctly.

Your food can boost your immune system, or it can totally tank it. You choose.

If you're looking for a down-and-dirty recommendation from me as to how to begin addressing your specific food choices, I'd say to reduce or remove grains, dairy, sugar, and processed foods. Focus on eating real foods, the way they were grown. For example: eat an apple, not an apple fruit snack. Eat a bowl of homemade rolled oats, not a granola cereal bar. Keep things simple and natural. And by the way—if you really want to accelerate your results, I'd say go "ALL IN!" I'd commit to stopping all grains, dairy, sugar, and alcohol for at least five weeks. I know you'll be glad you did! I challenge you to try it (and also focus on the mindset and other lifestyle recommendations) and then report back to me with how it went. I can't even wait to hear your success story. I'm rooting you on from afar!

The reasoning behind these food choices is because most people do have a tough time digesting grains and dairy, which causes stress and consequent inflammation in their body. Sugar is never beneficial, and processed foods are generally loaded with pretty inflammatory ingredients. If you're reading this book, I know there's something in your own health that you'd love to improve, whether that's more restful sleep, more energy, or the reversal of a long-standing autoimmune condition or disease. Your body is already under stress and depleted of its natural energy, and if we can do it a favor by reducing these foods, it can finally begin to heal within—which will make it easier for it to do its job.

By eliminating all four for a period of time—sugar, grains, dairy, and processed foods—you "clear the muddy water" in your body, so to speak. The chaos that can result internally from these offenders will be cleared up, and you can then start to see what's *really* going on and you'll start feeling better in ways you never imagined. Taking out these foods is a great place to start in order to reduce the amount of inflammation in your system and thereby allow your body more energy to rebalance and calibrate. If you still have other food intolerances beyond these, the reduced amount of inflammation in your system due to taking these out will at least help. Then you'll fine-tune as you go! Less inflammation from food = WINS.

CONSTIPATION

As we've discussed, constipation happens when food spends too much time in the large intestine, and too much liquid is soaked up from the digested food. It can occur because of dehydration, stress, or lack of exercise, and it could even be solved on its own if daily water intake is increased and fibrous foods are consumed. However, that's not always the case.

Constipation can also happen as a symptom of intestine inflammation. If a virus or another bacteria is in the digestive system, inflammation occurs as a defensive response. This can temporarily paralyze the stomach and intestines, bringing the digestive processes to a halt, which means the digested food is in the large intestine for far longer than it should be, losing more and more water to the colon's absorption.

To get things moving again, hydration is a great place to start—in addition to following all the anti-inflammation tips in this book if you're experiencing it chronically. Add more fibrous foods into your diet such as leafy vegetables, and also try some light exercise.

Most of all, though, don't just dose up on laxatives or "detox teas." You really need to address the root cause of it once and for all. Yes, you've "always been this way," but it's time you change that story.

DIARRHEA

We've learned that diarrhea occurs in irritable bowel syndrome when the large intestine contracts too quickly, hurrying the digested food along without properly absorbing all of the liquids. But there are many other reasons why diarrhea can occur. If the small intestine realizes that the food has bad bacteria or that a virus has entered your system, it will work to rid your body of the contaminated digested food as quickly as possible. Since it doesn't want to absorb any of the nutrients in the contaminated substance, movement through the small intestine and large intestine happens very quickly, leading to the watery diarrhea. It's your body's way of protecting you as quickly as possible.

Diarrhea also happens from inflammation. If the walls of your intestine are inflamed, they can't absorb nutrients and may be more easily irritated by what you've eaten. So, the muscles of the large intestine contract quickly to rid the system of the waste, since the digestive system isn't working properly.

If diarrhea becomes chronic or lasts for longer than a few days, it can be quite dehydrating. The best ways to help your body temporarily while you fix the underlying root causes include increasing water intake and staying away from dehydrators like caffeine and alcohol.

What if diarrhea may not be due to contaminated foods at all? What if it's due to a food intolerance? Or, what if food isn't even related to the cause, and the root of your digestive woes stems from your busy daily schedule and heightened mental stress? You absolutely must look closer to assess why this is really happening, and reverse the core imbalances in your mind, body, and environment.

GUT DYSBIOSIS

We talked a bit about gut dysbiosis in the chapter on joint and muscle inflammation. It occurs when the microbiota, or the composition of bacteria in the gut, has an unhealthy balance between the good bacteria, bad bacteria, and overall environment. Dysbiosis points to an imbalance in your gut that prevents your digestive system from working as it should.

Every day we are exposed to situations that may cause our gut to lose its balance and harmony, and therefore create this unhealthy state of dysbiosis. But why is it that some people's bodies experience symptoms, and others are just fine? Well, bad bacteria can unleash their danger when the internal environment of your digestive system is subpar.

QUICK CHECKLIST

You may have gut dysbiosis if:

❏ You experience inflammation in any way.
Gut dysbiosis can lead to joint inflammation,
psychological stress and mental disorders,
digestive inflammation, acne, and more. It's always
worth a look at your gut if you're experiencing any
health problems.

Here's another way to think about it: imagine that you order groceries, but you don't hear the doorbell and completely forget that you ordered them. So, you go about your day, go to sleep, and don't notice the groceries sitting on your doorstep until the next day. If you ordered raw chicken and it's been sitting in the heat outside your house for twenty-four hours, it's a probable bet that it's now covered in bad bacteria, and I would absolutely not take the risk of eating it. The hot environment outside made it so that the chicken was in an environment conducive to bacterial growth and contamination.

Contrast this with if you did hear the doorbell and immediately placed the raw chicken in your fridge. Since it stayed cold and fresh, it didn't experience any type of bacterial growth. It was in the proper environment to stay well. The environment matters for whether or not bad bacteria can grow and stay populated within your own body, which is why taking a holistic approach to your health and making sure you're doing everything you can to lessen stressors that may lead to intestinal inflammation is paramount for keeping your microbiota in a healthy homeostasis. Simply put, a truly healthy body will not be able to host bad things. If the internal body environment is healed, the rest of your body functions can fully activate and thrive.

Gut dysbiosis can lead to a host of problems: joint inflammation, psychological stress and mental disorders, digestive inflammation, acne . . . the balancing of the gut matters a great deal for the overall homeostasis of the body. That's why it's so important to get the balancing of the gut under control. If you suspect that you have too much bad bacteria or a parasite in your gut, the only way to know for sure is to find a functional medicine practitioner and have comprehensive testing completed. Ask your practitioner to look into this testing for you, and you can also visit my website at www.maggieberghoff.com to see my recommended steps for working with someone virtually or online who can do this for you.

SOLVING MARCY'S DIGESTIVE SYMPTOMS

When Marcy and I began to work together, we uncovered a number of reasons that she was experiencing these painful and uncomfortable digestive symptoms. For one, a great number of bacteria, heavy metals, and parasites had built up in her gut, so she was experiencing gut dysbiosis. We got to work detoxing her gently on a daily basis through various lifestyle means, giving her a very specific, individualized, yet simple plan to follow to begin her rebalancing process. We also began a targeted supplementation regimen to help her body heal the gut lining and supply her with the nutrients she needs.

We also recognized that the stress from the pressures of her job and its corresponding travel schedule had been taking a toll on her. So we created a new way to approach work that would reduce her stress levels. This didn't require fewer hours or backing off from excelling in her job; rather, we rearranged some things to help her thrive and become even more productive without the stress. By slowing down in certain areas of her life and balancing her high-stress career with stress-reducing techniques, she actually was able to accomplish even more at work, and reported a minimum of two hours MORE full energy during each workday, where she was laser-focused and productive without brain fog, fatigue, or headaches interfering. She was motivated and genuinely happy again.

We are all able to manage stress without sacrificing our careers or stepping back at work, and making these changes enables us to do even *better* at our jobs—while feeling better, too! The last thing we did for Marcy was to clear up toxins in her home and office environment thanks to a high-quality water filtration system and an air filtration system. We also cleaned up the products she was using in her home and office to lessen toxicities burdening her health and energy. These were simple, easy swaps that each made a massive difference. Reducing her Total Toxic Burden worked! Her digestive symptoms were completely alleviated once the inflammation went down. And the fatigue, brain fog, sleepless nights, and anxiety also went away, revealing a more powerful, happy, and healthy Marcy— ready to conquer her days again!

According to research, psychological stress has long been reported as a connection to IBS.[3] When you're stressed, your entire body feels it—which is why you may feel like your digestive system starts to act up when you're preparing for a big work meeting or coping with stress at home. And, as we learned in chapter 6, this gut inflammation and dysbiosis can lead to symptoms of depression, anxiety, and negative thoughts, thus propagating the vicious cycle of stress since the gut is attached to the brain. Stress can both cause digestive symptoms and be caused *by* gut problems. It's all interconnected. By reducing inflammatory stressors, everything in your body can be brought back to homeostasis, restoring and healing your gut lining, digestive inflammation, and the uncomfortable symptoms associated with common digestive conditions.

As you learn more about all the different types of inflammation symptoms and causes, I hope you start to see how interconnected the body is. We can't talk about one system without discussing another. The body functions in unison, and we must heal it as such as well. There are countless benefits of reducing inflammatory stressors, and this can have long-reaching implications for your health and wellness. For example: if you've been struggling with digestive symptoms but have never felt aches and pains in your joints, shifting your diet and balancing your gut bacteria can prevent you from ever having that joint inflammation. When inflammation goes down, your entire body—and your holistic health—benefits.

ALLERGIES, ASTHMA, AND SKIN INFLAMMATION

t's a beautiful spring afternoon and you're walking your dog through the park near your neighborhood. Flowers are blooming, the sun is shining, the breeze is just right—a truly perfect day! And then, it happens: the wind picks up pollen from the garden, and you start sneezing, uncontrollably. One violent sneeze after another, in tandem with the uncomfortable nose itchiness, eyes watering, and that itchy tingle in your throat. You have to move off to the side of the park's trail to recuperate. Does this sound like you or someone you know? Or, possibly your seasonal allergies lead to very scary symptoms such as dizziness or vertigo.

QUICK CHECKLIST

You may have allergies if:

❑ Your eyes are red, swollen, itchy, and puffy, making you want to wear big dark sunglasses!

❑ You have a case of the sniffles, but the itchy, annoying type.

❏ You can't stop sneezing, and it's getting disruptive.
❏ You go through too many packs of tissues to count.
❏ You feel tickles in the back of your throat that prompt you to cough.

Seasonal allergies are most commonly caused by pollen and are also referred to as "hay fever." Both the lining of your nose and your eyes swell and become inflamed in response to the allergens, which leads to all the sneezing and eyes watering. For some, allergy season means a stuffy nose all spring long, thanks to the congestion from nose-lining inflammation.

This visceral itchy, sneezing response doesn't come only from allergy season and its corresponding pollen and allergens floating through the wind. It can also come from inside your house, meaning you're constantly exposed to allergens and irritants like pet dander, household dust from your shoes, chemical odors from paints and adhesives, and even fragrances, like your hand soap or favorite perfume, all within the comfort and "safety" of your own home.

Allergies refer to your body's response to the irritants, and what is an irritant to you may differ greatly from what's an irritant to someone else. Allergies are simply your body's response to a foreign substance or pathogen, which is usually an overreaction on the part of the immune system. Suspecting danger—even if it's from a getaway fluff of your friend's cat's fur—the immune system kicks into high gear to produce antibodies to attack the trigger. It does this through the release of a chemical called a "histamine," which is responsible for all the swelling and the itching.

You have seen and have likely used antihistamines such as Claritin and Zyrtec, which provide relief from the symptoms of the body's histamine release. While, as with rescue inhalers, it's great to have medications like these to help stop all the sneezing and discomfort, it's still only masking the problem. Understanding that the body is reacting to these allergens and irritants and thus causing the allergy symptoms in response to them is crucial. The only real way to eliminate or alleviate allergies is to decrease the number of allergens your body is exposed to and build up your immune system to be able to better handle certain offenders, lessening or even completely eliminating your allergies.

I know, I know. This seems almost impossible—especially in the springtime, when common pollen and dander allergens are constantly floating through the air. The truth is, you can't control the irritants and stressors that you'll come into contact with when you have a picnic in the park or even walk past your neighbors' pesticide-covered weeds on your way to the mailbox. Even air pollution from cars or factory fumes in the air can cause inflammation. This doesn't mean you should avoid going outside. Please don't coop up in your home for fear of toxins or illness; it will only make you worse physically and mentally.

Rather, addressing environmental inflammation is about focusing on what you *can* control: the irritants and allergens in your house, in your bedroom, and in your workspace. By controlling these stressors, your body is far more equipped to handle the outside stressors you're exposed to the moment you walk out of your house, because it's not constantly reacting to irritants while you're sleeping in a dander-filled bedroom or cooking in a toxic chemical–sprayed kitchen. It's also about boosting your immune system. A strong immune system can tackle just about anything that comes its way. We'll dive into great depth on how to create an environment that sets you up for success in Step Three.

ASTHMA

When you have asthma, the lining of your airways becomes inflamed because of an irritant. This leads to the sense that it's hard to get a full breath, which causes wheezing, a fast heart rate, and a great deal of discomfort from chest tightness and the shortness of breath. The list of potential asthma triggers is extensive: pollen, pet hair, dust mites, tobacco smoke, heartburn, dander, and chemical fragrances. Triggers can also include exercise, stress, strong emotions, and hormone fluctuations. Asthma can happen as a result of allergies, or on its own.

QUICK CHECKLIST

You may have asthma if:

- ❏ It's difficult to get a full breath, as if your lungs feel heavy or blocked.
- ❏ Breathing in or out sharply creates a wheezing sound.
- ❏ You become lightheaded frequently from being unable to breathe.

These irritants lead to the swelling and inflammation of the lungs and airways. When someone is having an asthma attack or begins to experience the uncomfortable symptoms associated with asthma, the first rule of thumb is to use a rescue inhaler, most commonly with a bronchodilator called albuterol. It works by relaxing the muscles of the lungs, which dissipates the symptoms. Although rescue inhalers truly do come to the rescue in breathless moments, they work solely as Band-Aids. The inhalers do not prevent the asthmatic symptoms from happening again. Without addressing the environmental factors that cause asthma and asthma attacks, it's only a matter of time until the lungs and airways become inflamed once again from the same irritants that caused them to swell the first time.

CHRONIC SKIN INFLAMMATION

When skin inflammation occurs, it's almost always because of an imbalance in your body's internal environment—unless you apply a lotion that you're allergic to, or have some type of reaction to something else that's applied directly to your skin. In this chapter, we'll survey some of the most common skin conditions that I see (psoriasis, acne, and eczema), as well as uncomfortable skin symptoms such as hives, rashes, itchiness, and dry spots.

QUICK CHECKLIST

You may have chronic skin inflammation if:

- ❏ The skin appears red and inflamed.
- ❏ Skin is uncomfortably itchy or has a burning sensation.
- ❏ The skin becomes raw or cracked.
- ❏ The skin appears to thicken.
- ❏ There are blisters or acne on the skin.

Skin is the body's largest organ, and because of its connection to every system within the body, it can provide evidence as to an internal imbalance that's occurring. If you experience chronic hives, frequent rashes, dry and itchy patches, or can't seem to clear up your acne no matter how many high-quality skin cleansers you try, there's definitely something going on internally. When something is wrong with the body, it acts out—and can act out on your skin, specifically.

PSORIASIS

Celine came to me with psoriasis: a skin condition marked by itchy, dry patches that can be red, covered with silvery scales, and feel as though they're "burning." Psoriasis is thought to be a chronic skin condition that flares up in cycles. For Celine, she would think that it was finally cleared up, then the symptoms would frustratingly come back time and time again.

QUICK CHECKLIST

You may have psoriasis if:

❏ Your skin becomes red or patchy, with scales.
❏ Your skin is itchy, feels like it's burning, or is sore.
❏ Alongside your skin symptoms, your joints feel stiff.
❏ Nails may become thickened or rough.

The cause of psoriasis has never been officially determined, but it's thought to be caused by the immune system. In psoriasis, the body's T cells attack healthy skin cells, leading to the dry, itchy, red patches marked by psoriasis. There are several types of psoriasis depending on where on your body you're experiencing it: plaque psoriasis on the skin; nail psoriasis, which affects the fingers and toenails; pustular psoriasis, which occurs on the hands, feet, and fingertips; and the less common erythrodermic psoriasis, which can cover the entire body.

Additionally, psoriatic arthritis can occur, which couples the dry and itchy skin patches with joint inflammation and arthritis symptoms. As we'll learn in this chapter, skin symptoms and conditions are also caused by problems that happen within the body.

Celine had tried topical steroids and medications in an attempt to clear up her psoriasis and restore relief to her skin. It never worked, or never provided relief for very long. Sometimes the steroids and medications would temporarily alleviate the symptoms, but they always came back. When she came to me for help, I knew immediately that we needed to look at her internal body environment. Once we did and addressed the potential imbalances, her skin returned to vibrant, glowing, clear health without the assistance of any steroids, topical creams, or medications. Almost like magic!

THE CONNECTION BETWEEN THE GUT AND THE SKIN

For Celine specifically, we looked at her gut. I suspected that there could be gut dysbiosis that was causing her psoriasis, so we got to work cleaning up the bad bacteria and promoting good bacteria in her gut lining. When I see skin inflammation and rashes, it's usually a symptom of yeast or candida overgrowth in the gut, or some other type of dysbiosis.

Candida and yeast overgrowth typically occur as the result of your diet. Consistently eating foods that are high in refined sugars, white flours, or have a lot of dairy or carbs can contribute to the overgrowth. Additionally, a high alcohol intake, a weakened immune system, and taking antibiotics and oral contraceptives can contribute.

In addition to resulting in skin and nail infections, candida overgrowth can also present as fatigue, frequent urinary tract infections and sinus infections, and digestive issues such as constipation and diarrhea. Now, the only way to know for sure if you have candida overgrowth in your gut is to abide by the gold standard and do testing. But, if you suspect that you have it, you can also start to improve it on your own through your diet and watching what you eat. Those white-flour, processed, high-sugar foods don't do you any favors! And, continuing to eat them contributes even more to an internal environment that is out of balance.

You could try an anti-candida diet, which consists of leafy greens, eggs, meat, nuts and seeds, and herbal tea, and remove foods such as sugar and many carbohydrates, and even fruit. However, remember that following a "diet" isn't going to heal you. Spinach and kale cannot magically heal you, despite our preconceptions about their mystical, health-inducing powers. What these whole foods *do* help to do is nourish the body and give it what it needs to heal itself, to start to rewire, and to rebuild. You need to look beyond food, as well. Why did the candida or gut dysbiosis happen in the first place? Are you mentally stressed and under a lot of pressure? Is your sleep disturbed? Find the root cause and address that in addition to making food changes.

Even if it's not candida overgrowth specifically that's playing a role in your skin inflammation, any type of gut dysbiosis can play a part. An article in *Frontiers of Microbiology* noted that "cumulative evidence has demonstrated an intimate, bidirectional connection between the gut and skin."[1] It went on to share research that "in cases of disturbed intestinal barriers, intestinal bacteria as well as intestinal microbiota metabolites have been reported to gain access to the bloodstream, accumulate in the skin, and disrupt skin homeostasis."[2] So, when bad bacteria accumulate in the gut or any type of imbalance occurs, it can easily access the skin, too, and cause problems! This can lead to psoriasis, acne, and other skin symptoms.

ACNE

Acne refers to the development of zits, pimples, whiteheads, blackheads—you name it, any type of growth on the skin as a result of the blockage or inflammation of the hair follicles. It's most commonly on the face, but it also can frequently develop on the back and on the chest. Research has explored the contributors to acne, and it once again has been traced back to the gut. Researchers Whitney P. Bowe and Alan C. Logan concluded in their study that "there appears to be more than enough supportive evidence to suggest that gut microbes, and the integrity of the gastrointestinal tract itself, are contributing factors in the acne process."[3]

QUICK CHECKLIST

You may have acne if:

❏ There are blemishes on your skin in the form of pimples, whiteheads, or blackheads.

Acne, like the other skin conditions, is also a result of a disruption in the body's internal homeostasis.

Of course, this goes back to diet once again. Those sugars, processed foods, and white carbohydrates certainly don't help, especially if you suspect candida overgrowth or have previously noticed a high sensitivity or an intolerance to these foods. And there's specific research that says high doses of dairy may contribute to acne. The study, titled "Dairy Intake and Acne Vulgaris," studied an analysis group of 78,529 individuals ranging in age from seven to thirty years old. "In conclusion, any dairy, such as milk, yogurt, and cheese, was associated with an increased OR [odds ratio] for acne in individuals aged 7–30 years," it noted.[4]

The study was not necessarily conclusive and had some limitations. So, it's not the case that if you ditch the ice cream, milk, and cheese your skin will immediately clear up. Again, these are nuanced recommendations and there's no one magic cure. Every single body is different, and some are more dairy sensitive than others. How I want you to think about this is not that there will be one fix that works across the board and for everyone. I wish that I could tell you, "Eliminate this and your acne will clear up," or "Add this to your diet and the acne will disappear." How easy that would be! It's never that simple, because it's a much more holistic process. Sometimes acne may even be due to your mindset, toxicities, or stress levels instead of your diet! Healing is about taking a closer look at factors that are going on not only in your gut but also in your environment along with any other stressors that may be impacting you. Again, we return to that Total Toxic Burden.

Maybe you notice that whenever you have an exam coming up, you break out. Or you're going through a stressful life period because you're switching to a new job or beginning your own company, and your skin is very visibly showing your stress! Stress can contribute in a serious way. Research from the University of Zagreb School of Medicine noted, "Even though emotional stress has long been suspected to trigger or exacerbate acne, its influence on acne severity has been mostly underestimated until recently when studies have brought new data about the different mechanisms and possible factors involved in this interaction."[5]

They went on to say that "this bidirectional intimate relationship of the skin and the mind emphasizes the importance of a holistic and interdisciplinary approach to caring for patients with acne," which I completely agree with. When working with a client experiencing chronic skin inflammation, this holistic approach is critical. In addition to cleaning up the gut, I urge you to evaluate what psychological stress you may be under—whether it's temporary because of something going on in your life right now or more chronic.

The good news is that clearing up your environment and living an anti-inflammatory lifestyle with the tools in this book can help to alleviate both stress and skin problems, as we learned in chapter 6 on psychological stress. Currently, there may be a war going on between your gut and a bacteria imbalance, its effect on your mind through the enteric nervous system, and your skin through both the stress and your gut! By taking a holistic approach and restoring balance to your whole body, many of your symptoms will likely clear up at once.

ECZEMA

Eczema is another skin inflammation condition in which the individual experiences an irritating, dry rash that can make the skin red, itchy, and "scaly" all over the body. There are several different types of eczema. The most common is called atopic dermatitis (AD), which is more severe and tends to be chronic. There is also specifically hand eczema, which affects the hand and wrist region. Eczema is most common in children, who can grow out of it as adults. But adults can develop it, too, even if they never had it as children.

QUICK CHECKLIST

You may have eczema if:

❑ Your skin is incredibly dry, no matter how much heavy-duty moisturizer you slather on.

❑ Your skin is red and itchy.

❑ Your skin appears to be scaly.

There is no specific medical "cure" for eczema—rather, those who have it will utilize treatments such as topical cortico-steroids, lotions, and other medications to seek relief. However, if we take a holistic view as to why the eczema is happening, we can usually help clear it up for good by eliminating the cause! SO—how to find the cause? Well, look at mental stress, your nutrition, products you're using on your body, and types of liquids you're drinking. Assess how you're breaking down and absorbing food—are your stools normal? Do you have any gut symptoms like bloating or constipation? A study from *Allergy, Asthma & Immunology Research* on the connection between the gut microbiome and atopic dermatitis found that "the gut microbiome may contribute to the development, persistence, and severity of AD via immunologic, metabolic, and neuroen-docrine pathways." It also noted, "Metagenomic analyses in humans and animals clearly demonstrated that AD is associ-ated with the dysbiosis of the gut and skin microbiome."[6]

HIVES

Hives is another skin problem, but rather than being a condi-tion itself, it is usually a symptom of another autoimmune condition or reaction to an imbalance in the body. Hives are either pale or red bumps that erupt from the skin, and are commonly very itchy or present a "burning" sensation. Of course, they often and commonly occur as the result of an allergy—such as if you're allergic to cats. Your immune system will react in the same part of your skin that touched the cat's fur, sending histamines to that area—which you'll remember from the environmental section of this chapter are the body's chemical response to some type of irritant. The histamines are sent to fight the "pathogen," which in this example is the cat's fur.

QUICK CHECKLIST

You may have hives if:

❏ You experience a series of tiny pale or red bumps
   on your skin.
❏ The bumps are very itchy or feel like they're
   burning.

The medical name for hives when they're chronic is "chronic urticaria." An article titled "Chronic Urticaria and Autoimmunity" reported that "over half of all cases of chronic idiopathic urticaria are thought to occur by an autoimmune mechanism."[7]

Most commonly, chronic hives are associated with thyroid disease and rheumatoid arthritis—autoimmune diseases we have discussed in this book already. Hives are caused by histamines regardless of whether they're caused by an allergy (like the contact with a cat's fur) or not. The histamines rush to what's being perceived as a threat, even if it's healthy tissue. Antihistamines are a common treatment, and while they may temporarily alleviate the hives, the hives will come back—it's just a matter of when! These Band-Aid "solutions" are not really solutions at all. We must find the cause of the overactive immune system and rebalance the body to be able to handle the offenders.

Whether you know which autoimmune condition you have or are experiencing hives for seemingly no reason, the solution to start with is going to be the same: reducing the number of stressors that the body is subjected to. By decreasing the stressors, inflammation and the body's immune system attacks will begin to decrease, too, returning the body to homeostasis.

RASHES

Rashes are yet another symptom of inflammation within the body. Defined as the temporary itchiness, redness, dryness, or sensitivity of skin, they're the result of an immune system reaction. If you've ever tried a lotion or a perfume that you were sensitive or allergic to, you likely developed a rash because the immune system rushed to the site of the harmful substance. This is, as I mentioned, one of the only reasons that a skin inflammation would occur as the result of something outside of the body. If you have rashes but didn't use any products that could cause the reaction, it's the result of something internal.

QUICK CHECKLIST

You may have rashes if:

❏ There is a patch or several patches of redness and irritation on your skin.
❏ There are patches of dryness.
❏ There are skin patches where the skin is particularly sensitive.

Rashes are usually symptoms of another disorder: rheumatoid arthritis, psoriasis, eczema, or thyroid disease. Regardless of what specifically caused the rash, the important next step is to eliminate stressors and help the body return to balance. A rash—and any other skin inflammation—is your body's way of speaking up. It's evidence that something isn't quite right. It's a call for help that requires a holistic look at your diet, gut, environment, mindset, and anything else that can be contributing to the imbalance within you that's causing your immune system to act up.

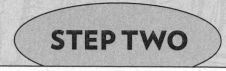

STEP TWO

AN ANTI-INFLAMMATORY WAY OF LIFE

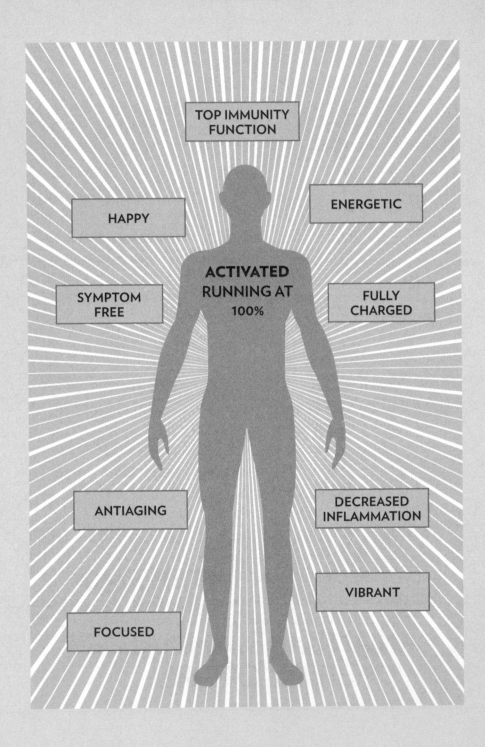

9

MINDSET AND MINDFULNESS

When I first started working with private clients, I typically would begin by discussing one thing in particular: cleaning up their environment. We are going to dive deep into the most common environmental stressors and how to fix them in chapter 10—but as important and crucial as all those steps are, I realized from my experience with these clients that the *most* fundamental aspect of healing is actually *mindset* first and foremost. In fact, if mindset wasn't tackled first, nothing else moved the needle forward in the client's health. Your mindset is the single most important factor toward living a life free from health struggles and full of abundance. Once mindset is on point, everything else can flow more easily.

We can clean up your environment, transform your diet, get you moving, and revamp your pantry, but if your headspace isn't where it needs to be, *healing will be slow or nonexistent*.

Dr. Joe Dispenza is an author and thought leader who preaches the power of the mind and meditation to heal the body. His belief in our ability to transform our bodies through our minds began with his own experience. In 1986, he was participating in a triathlon and was hit by a car when he was on his bike. The crash shattered his spine. The doctors told him it was

127

unlikely he would ever walk again unless he underwent a risky surgical procedure that could take his life.[1]

So he decided to take matters into his own hands. He left the hospital despite the doctor's warning against it. He meditated, or "went within," every day for two hours and meditated on the belief that his spine was healing on its own. He saw a totally healed spine in his mind's eye and imagined walking again with ease.

Only *nine and a half weeks* later, his spine was healed and he was able to walk. Now, this was entirely without any type of surgery or body cast. Today he helps people around the world understand the profound connection of their minds and bodies, and in addition to his own story, he has countless client and reader testimonials of similar "miracles." And you know how much I love a good miracle!

In one of his most famous books, *Breaking the Habit of Being Yourself*, Dispenza shares information on an experiment done by Glen Rein, PhD, a cellular biologist.[2] The study was conducted at the HeartMath Research Center in California, which was studying how our emotions impact our heart's functionality and the regularity of its beats. When we're angry, stressed, or sad, our hearts actually beat erratically and in a disorganized rhythm. But when we're happy and feeling joyful and full of appreciation, our heartbeats find a coherent rhythm. We need this coherence for optimal health and healing.

In the experiment, Dr. Rein used trained HeartMath participants who learned how to elevate their emotional state to love, joy, and appreciation. They then each held vials of DNA. The first group was supposed to feel this elevated emotion of love and joy while holding the vials. The second group was supposed to hold both the elevated emotion *and* a clear intention to either wind or unwind the DNA in the vial. The third group was instructed *not* to enter an elevated emotional state, and instead just focus their intention on winding or unwinding the DNA.

For the first and the third group, there were no statistically significant changes to the DNA in the vial. But for the second group—who held both an elevated emotion and an intention to change the DNA—the DNA was either wound or unwound (depending on the intention) as much as *25 percent*.

As you begin to embrace healing and the real techniques and strategies that have helped to heal so many of my clients, I need you to know how powerful your mind is. Your mind is where your emotions are born, and your mind is where you can choose to believe—or not believe—that your healing process is working. But you need both. You need to be in an elevated state of emotion AND you need to intend that changes are happening in your life. You need to will it with your own intention. I can't do that part for you, as much as I wish I could!

If you only half believe that there's no way you can heal because of your genetics, because several doctors have called your diagnosis incurable and lifelong, or because you have fallen into the belief that you have to experience these symptoms forever, you will experience what you believe (even if it's a half belief!), and you're right, you probably won't get better. Your body can only achieve what your mind believes, and once you put your mind toward something and truly embrace the growth, amazing things can happen.

We often think of DNA as unchangeable. After all, it's our DNA. It carries an imprint from our families and those who have come before us—especially for genetic conditions. But if you still have that belief within you—that DNA is unchanging and there's nothing you can do to really heal yourself—please read the study from HeartMath one more time. You can even heal DNA that *isn't yours*! If an elevated emotion and clear intention can change the DNA composition in a vial that's being held, imagine how an elevated emotion and clear intention can change the DNA composition that's in your body. This is the same with your food choices and the toxicities you're exposed to. You can change your DNA for the better, or you can change it for the worse. That choice is really up to you—you have the power to choose what you want and what you will change.

ALLEVIATING MENTAL STRESS

It is critical to find ways to alleviate stress in your life—especially now. Life is so go-go-go nowadays with more political and global turmoil than ever. The news bombards us with terrifying statistics and troubling stories that can send our minds into a tailspin after skimming one headline. Comparison is at an all-time high with social media putting unrealistic pressure on us to look or behave a certain way that we see on the "highlight reels" of most accounts. The world is moving FAST, and our bosses expect us to keep up with that pace and always go faster, harder, better. Even our little kids' schooling is getting more and more strict and demanding every day on not just them but also us as parents. No wonder so many of us are walking around at a baseline of "stressed"!

Alleviating this stress is more important than ever right now. Even if you do try to hold an elevated state of joy and you have a clear intention to heal, if stress is impacting you because of a busy week at work, a worry about a situation in your life, or even happy stress about an upcoming promotion or vacation, *your body will feel it inside.*

Mental stress is seldom talked about between patients and health professionals, and it's an important piece of the puzzle that's too often overlooked. Your nurse or doctor may briefly ask on an intake form or at the start of a visit what your "stress level" is and mark a tick in their notes of what you reported, but the conversation typically ends there. A report from the *Journal of the National Medical Association* surveyed 151 healthcare providers and reported that "forty-two percent of respondents reported receiving no instruction regarding stress and health outcomes during their medical/professional education. While 90% believed stress management was 'very' or 'somewhat' effective in improving health outcomes, 45% 'rarely' or 'never' discussed stress management with their patients."[3] They might mention in passing that you should "decrease your stress"—but that's really about the extent of it, which is a terrible disservice. That's like saying, "Just be happy," or "Don't worry." It does nothing to fix the problem. And further, if your practitioner *doesn't fully believe* you can heal, or if they don't believe in the power of the connection between the mind and the body, it will be so much harder for you to actually heal. It takes a great client-practitioner relationship where both parties fully believe in the ability you have within you to reach your health goals.

The lack of attention to stress is so concerning because stress is one of the *top indicators* of health and body homeostasis (or a lack thereof). Stress moves the body into a sympathetic nervous state. In this state, the body is ready to either fight or flee. It's the fight-or-flight state, and to prepare for the worst, the body floods with hormones that cause a rush of blood flow to the skin and muscles and an increase in heart rate. You could be operating from this inflammation-ridden sympathetic nervous system all day, every day—and not fully know it!

As long as you're in the sympathetic nervous system, it doesn't matter what we clear up. You could be on the world's cleanest, most nutritious diet, breathing in the freshest air, and drinking nontoxic water, and still experience every single one of your symptoms because you're stuck in a constant sympathetic nervous state. Without the strategies and tools to bring you out of that state from time to time, the body won't be able to find a balance. There are a lot of strategies that will help to get your body out of a sympathetic nervous state. Of course, you can take things off your plate, slow down, be real with yourself on how fast you really "need" to go and where you may need to think about slowing down or bringing in help. Maybe you can hire a team member? Reduce hours at work or switch into a different role? Hire help around the home to get things done and make life easier on you?

Other techniques that can help you to manage stress could be red-light therapy, grounding, and breath work—as you'll learn about in later sections. With these tools, you can absolutely live in this modern life *without* overstressing or burning out your body. In fact, when your mindset is on point and your internal body is balanced, you will be even more productive, energetic, and efficient, achieving *more* while feeling better. It's absolutely possible!

The goal is to activate the parasympathetic nervous state, which is what you need to learn to be able to activate yourself if you're going to see positive changes in your health. The parasympathetic nervous system calms the body down, and it's also optimal for healing. It makes sure the body is balanced and in a state to heal and regenerate. Think about it this way: if you were being chased by a mountain lion, would your body care at all about regulating your temperature, heart rate, and digestion? Likely, no. There are far bigger (and scarier) issues to attend to in that moment—you are in survival mode only.

Your body constantly sets off that same exact reaction of "survival mode" in today's world, which is where the major problem lies. You may be activating a sympathetic nervous state due to a looming deadline, worry over a simple decision you have to make, the irritation of being stuck in traffic, or the frustration of a long wait for a customer service call. The body was not made to be in fight-or-flight mode for long periods of time, or for that to be activated for something that isn't life-threatening. Rather, this was supposed to be a reserve for moments of danger.

By engaging the parasympathetic nervous system, you bring your body back to balance, and help it to heal. To do this, make sure you are always checking in with your breath. When stressed, our breathing tends to be quick and shallow, or we may even be holding our breath while reading that email or fighting feelings of irritation at the long line in the grocery store. These are optimal moments to insert the breath, to tell the body everything is OK. Sometimes, it might not immediately come to mind that you should focus on your breath. So, if you're going through a period in which you're more stressed than usual, set some timers in your phone to go off every hour as a reminder to unclench your jaw and focus on your breathing.

HOW TO BREATHE

What can you do that is 1) free; 2) so easy; 3) no one will ever notice you're doing it, so it can be used in the EXACT moment of heightened stress? BREATHE.

Through a certain way of breathing, you can activate your parasympathetic nervous system almost immediately and get out of the sympathetic fight-or-flight mode. It's quick, effective, and free.

Do this exercise, right now.

First, pick a color. Your favorite, most peaceful color. The color that makes you feel comfortable and home. Do you have it?

Now close your eyes. With this in mind, breathe in through your nose for four seconds. Hold your breath for four seconds, then exhale for four seconds. Hold again, for four seconds. Repeat slowly, three to five more times. Truly think about your breath. Think about the air going in and out of your nose on the "one . . . two . . . three . . . four" as you gracefully time your inhale and exhale. Think about your body filling up with that favorite and most peaceful color. Think of the color coming in and circling peacefully around every part of your body, head to toe. Think of your body sinking into a state of calmness. Allow all the stress and worry to fully leave your body on every exhale. Allow joy and happiness to enter on every inhale.

If you're in traffic or in the middle of a meeting and the stress creeps in and your heart and mind start racing, you can do this exact thing with your eyes open.

This technique can calm you at any given time—it's even very helpful before meals to prepare the digestive system for breaking down and absorbing food, and before bed to calm the body and prepare for restful sleep. There's honestly not a single time of the day when it isn't helpful! So, even if you're reading this book right now, whether you're "zenned out" on a hammock or in the bathtub with the most relaxing cup of tea in the world, take a minute to try this with me. Do just a few minutes of this breathing technique and sink into an even more peaceful state.

Every day, prioritize spending just a few minutes to engage the parasympathetic nervous system through this breathing technique.

VISUALIZATION

Just as the research from the HeartMath Institute suggests, visualization can be deeply and profoundly transformational for our bodies. If simply setting an intention while holding vials of DNA can unwind DNA by up to 25 percent, imagine what daily visualization can do for our bodies! There are two visualization practices that I live by, which you can use on an as-needed basis. However, I do strongly encourage you to make visualization a daily practice. Many of my clients enjoy visualizing first thing in the morning. Just a few minutes for these exercises with your morning cup of matcha or lemon water will go a long way. Really feel the gratitude and peace of each of these visualizations.

VISUALIZING YOURSELF IN VIBRANT HEALTH

If there is a health goal that you have—even if it's just recovering and living a life free of aches and pains—set aside some time to visualize and really feel how it would be if you were in truly vibrant health. Imagine what you would do, the feelings of gratitude and excitement, and whatever comes up for you. The longer you can linger in this "mind movie," the better! It will get you excited about the health freedom that is coming your way. It may seem like "daydreaming," as it should! Allow your mind to explore just how good it can really be. This is helping more than you know, because when we imagine something with a high level of emotion or excitement attached to it, we're more likely to bring it into our experience.

VISUALIZING NUTRIENTS IN THEIR FULL POWER

One of my own favorite forms of visualization is something you can do after or while you eat a meal. Really think about that nutrient-rich, colorful, and healthy meal with everything in it that your body needs to be strong and healthy. Because I eat for fuel, I put extra attention on how every bite and ingredient is helping my body! Here's how you can be really intentional about this in your visualization:

1. While you're eating, take a few minutes to close your eyes and take a few deep breaths.
2. Think through each of the vegetables, seeds, nuts, and proteins that you have just consumed or that you are current consuming, one by one.
3. Imagine that all of the nutrients from each food are swimming to every cell in your body, filling them with everything your body needs to recuperate and be strong and vibrant. Your body is so happy and is sending you many thanks for such a great import of nutrients today!
4. Slow down and "see" your food. Rather than gulping down a smoothie on your way out the door, take smaller, more intentional sips and think about every ingredient you thoughtfully placed into the blender. Commend your choices to use a nut milk to rebalance your body, as opposed to a sugar-laden fruit juice that would have slowed it down. Imagine every teaspoon of cacao powder or chia seeds and their anti-inflammatory powers. Do this as if you're a famous food critic trying each spice and each herb of a restaurant's famous dish, or like a wine sommelier who really spends time with each sip of wine to get all of its notes and tannins. Psst . . . this is also a great mindfulness exercise!
5. Fast-forward, mentally, to tomorrow, when all your cells have taken in all of the nutrients. Imagine how strong and energetic you will feel! Imagine how you will look physically—in your face and smile—with a body shining bright happy energy from it.
6. Zoom out and imagine your body in one week, one month, and one year as you continue to feed it good, whole foods with anti-inflammatory and antioxidant properties. Visualize how your body will feel and

the energy that will be available to you! Your cells say THANK YOU for the wonderful gift of the nutrients you have given them.

GRATITUDE

One of the simplest things we can do daily to improve our mindset is to practice gratitude. I know, I know . . . we hear it all the time. But I'd be remiss to not mention it in this book, because gratitude is how we send a love letter to every cell of our body and every second of our experience. And it can truly work wonders. Yet many of us don't take time beyond superficially thinking, "Oh, yes, I am grateful." When we're in the midst of a hectic day, it can be hard to remember to slow down and find time to be still, grateful, and calm while we're running a million miles a minute and can hardly remember that our cup of tea is still in the microwave! It's too easy to be looking toward the next to-do-list item the minute we finish the current one. However, if we hit a personal "pause" button in the middle of even our busiest days—even for just sixty seconds of gratitude to put a smile on our face and elevate our mood—it can help our productivity, internal body chemistry, and overall health significantly.

I recommend thinking of three things in your life that you're grateful for every single morning, while you're still snuggled in bed, right before you get up. Don't worry, this won't take long. Thirty seconds tops! Usually when our alarms go off, we immediately try to get our bearings and remember what day it is and what's on our to-do lists. Or worse, our mind instantly goes to a place of worry, anxiety, or the negativity of "I don't want to get up . . . ," "I hate my job . . . ," "Is it Friday yet?!" and so forth. Those negative thoughts immediately put our body and mind in a terrible space—one that isn't conducive to health and vitality. And frankly, it gets the day off on the worst possible foot.

Think of that phrase, "Woke up on the wrong side of the bed." Any morning that doesn't begin with gratitude is a morning when you've woken up on the wrong side of the bed! Instead, I want you to wake up on the *right* side and consciously think through three things—and I encourage you to switch them up daily, so you don't just go through the motions (i.e., "my family, my friends, my house, OK let's go!") and instead, you can really *feel* the gratitude. It can be for something as simple as the warm sunrays coming through the shades, the sounds of the birds chirping this morning, or even that new shampoo that you're eager to try out in your morning shower!

The truth is, we have so much to appreciate that we often overlook because we've come to take it for granted. No matter what is going on in your life right now—what hardships or setbacks you've faced—I know with certainty there is a reason for you to be grateful and appreciative of *something*. Even as you're reading this book—have you taken a moment to appreciate the fact that you CAN read, and for that, you're able to lose an afternoon in a good book or educate yourself? Did you know that still, in 2020, about 10% of the world's population *cannot* read?[4]

Challenge yourself to feel gratitude for that which you usually take for granted. Feel it for each tasty sip of your matcha latte in the morning, for each giggle you share with your toddler, for each moment of comfort and relaxation when you sink a little deeper into your pillow at the end of a long day.

TIME IN NATURE

Time in nature is something that helps decrease inflammation tremendously. It helps to regulate circadian rhythm, aid our cortisol levels, provide fresh air, activate our parasympathetic state, and allow for a break. In fact, a study by Alan Ewert and

Yun Chang showed that just visiting natural locations (like walking through a park or going down to the beach) has been proven to be beneficial in reducing physical and psychological stress levels. They wrote that "visitors to a natural environment report[ed] significantly lower levels of stress than their counterparts [who visited] a more urbanized outdoor setting or indoor exercise facility." There's nothing better than some time outside to get away from the hustle and bustle and practice some more gratitude. Depending on where you live, take a walk out into the woods, walk along the ocean, take a stroll by a neighboring lake, or just sit in the grass among the flowers in your backyard or at a nearby park. However you can get away from the distractions of hectic everyday life, do it. This is so grounding and will help you connect with yourself on a deeper level. And, as you survey Mother Nature, I encourage you to feel gratitude for every bursting pink flower, every salty drop in the ocean, every pleasant breeze of wind, and every sunray that feels so good on your skin. You can even talk to nature, and "thank" every little item around you for being present. I know this sounds silly, but thanking the sky, the trees, the grass, the air, and the flowers and letting them know *why* you're thanking them will help you to heal. This mindfulness and gratitude practice is so easy to implement—for powerful results.

YOUR FRIENDS AND COMMUNITY

It's also crucial to survey who you're spending time with. I encourage you to align yourself with people who represent who you are becoming—people who act with love toward themselves, who make healthy choices, and who embody what you want to be. Maybe it's a community of people who run successful businesses but do it with grace and ease and prioritize time with family and time for health. Maybe it's a community of people who make the choice to minimize processed foods, grains, sugar, and dairy and prioritize meditation, exercise, creativity, and spirituality. One thing is for sure: as you undergo transformation, you cannot still spend time with people who aren't aligned with what you are becoming. I'm not telling you to ditch your lifelong friends or move cities to find a new crew. Rather, I want you to become hyperconscious of how everything and everyone you spend time with impacts your energy, and therefore your health and your life. We tend to revert to our old selves when we're with friends who align with that old self. You can still have love and gratitude for these friendships while opting to spend more time with people who align with your highest vision for yourself.

Hand in hand with this is simply imagining that you are already what you want to become. Imagine that you have become the most centered, joyful, peaceful, and healthy version of yourself. What does this new you do? What thoughts fill your headspace? How do you treat your body, and how do you treat others? What are the days filled with? The more you can step into this version—even if it's just via imagination—the more your intention to become this new you will catapult you toward the reality that you *are* the new you.

No matter what it is that you want to change—where you live, your relationship, your body composition, a disease, your career, cancer—*anything* is possible if you can get your mindset to truly believe and achieve it. I want to remind you that the mindset of being stuck where you are is a *choice*, and you get to choose every single day whether you'll believe in the new you or stay stuck in the old. If you keep telling yourself a story that keeps you stuck, such as blaming your health and condition on your genetics, saying you could "never" achieve or obtain that goal or that picture of health . . . Well, whatever lie you're telling yourself *is a lie*. The danger is when you've recited the lie so many times that you believe it to your core. If that's the case, you'll stay stuck in that "poor me" mentality for the rest of your life.

There is nothing stopping you, right now, from making a commitment to yourself to change your mentality. It can seem daunting to make many changes at once, but as you shift your diet in the next chapter and your environment in the chapter after that, consider that these changes will also serve as reminders of the new you that you are becoming. But the real work starts right here and now. Will you step up to the plate and show up for yourself? Will you practice an elevated state of emotions whenever possible? Will you have a clear intention for what you want for your life and your health? Will you believe with every bone in your body that you are destined for wellness and complete health? And if you don't yet fully believe, will you work on your mindset every single day to propel that belief?

It's up to you. If you're willing to make this foundational change, more health and happiness than you've ever known are available to you—*waiting* for you—on the other side of the transformation.

10

DETOXIFY AND OPTIMIZE YOUR HOME AND OFFICE ENVIRONMENT

One of the most important conversations around inflammation is how to decrease stress by addressing not just your psychological stress but your environmental stress as well. Aka a home detox! We've covered many of the systems that can be damaged greatly by inflammation, from the endocrine system to the digestive system. Now it's time to discuss WHERE that inflammation comes from in regard to your home environment. What caused it in your life? Why is your body reacting so negatively and feeling out of tune and out of balance? What is the root cause?

One place to look is your immediate environment: your air, water, food, light, and the products you use in your home or on your body. By understanding the most common stressors that affect us in our immediate environment, we can better understand what changes we must make to help our bodies rebalance and realign. Each of these stressors distracts our body's attention, taking valuable energy away from our body's natural processes. When we optimize them and create what I have termed "an environment to thrive," our body can decrease the stress it's under and heal.

My client Natalie came to me knowing already that she was experiencing inflammation from her environment, because she was simply so sensitive to it.

"When I walk into a friend's house, I can instantly tell if they have mold," she told me. She would immediately feel nauseated or could even get a migraine from the smell of chemicals. Because of her sensitivity, she was careful to live a nontoxic life: choosing only nontoxic makeup, hair care, and household products, and trying her best to stay away from anything that could incite the inflammation she was experiencing and its uncomfortable symptoms. Despite being extra diligent in staying away from these toxic problems, she was still constantly feeling nauseated or getting migraines. "What is it coming from?" she asked me, exasperated.

Addressing environmental stressors goes beyond just changing the products you use in your home. While it's certainly important to eliminate any toxic ingredients from your space (which, you betcha, we will take a good and hard look at), an assessment of environmental inflammation extends to the allergens in the air, pollutants outside, potential heavy metal toxicity in your tap water, sounds in your immediate environment, and even the light that you're exposed to.

This is all important to everyone—even those who don't sneeze up a storm every time spring comes around because of allergens in the air. We are all vulnerable to inflammation from stressors in our environment. By making the necessary adjustments to our environments, we decrease the total number of stressors impacting us, which keeps us below our Total Toxic Burden. This can alleviate a host of different symptoms and conditions, which is why I always assess a client's environment when helping them.

PART ONE:
OPTIMIZING YOUR ENVIRONMENT

PURIFYING YOUR AIR

For Natalie, we began to assess her environmental inflammation with a complete revamp of her home environment. This meant taking care of anything that would cause irritation. One thing we did for her was clean up the air in her home. Air purifiers are aptly named, as they work to purify the air in your home by pulling those airborne dust and pollen particles out of the air, then recirculating purified air.

It's my greatest recommendation to invest in an effective air purifier—and this recommendation is for *everyone*, not just those who have allergies or asthma. Every time you open your door, more dust, chemicals, bacteria, and pollen particles can enter your home. You bring them in on your shoes, and if you have dogs, they can bring in plenty of allergens from rolling in the grass and playing at the dog park. Even your own hair can trek pollen and allergens into the safety of your home. Thankfully, air purifiers take care of the purification for you, so you don't constantly have to worry about new irritants in the air.

Think of an air purifier as a vacuum cleaner. You can purchase one that will be transported from room to room, taking turns purifying the air in each room. If you don't yet have an air purifier, realize that every time you go to sleep at night, you're breathing in air with irritants that are affecting you. Dust mites from the unswept corners of your basement are coming up through the vents, pollen that became attached to your sweater during your walk yesterday is now airborne, and if you have pets, their dander is swirling around you, too. As you breathe while you sleep (or anytime you're at home doing anything!), you're inhaling these irritants, and your immune system is immediately getting to work to defend the body. No wonder chronic inflammation can occur!

I also recommend keeping air constantly circulating, which air purifiers certainly help with. You should also exchange the air volume in your home every day by simply opening windows in your house. Try to open windows in each room in your house or apartment at least three times a week to bring in that new, fresh, charged air, and circulate out the stagnant, stale air.

How often do you clean up your space? Aside from spring cleaning, I urge you to dust off your picture frames, sweep the floors, wipe down tables and desks, and keep your immediate environment tidy and clean. This will also help with the air in your home, because when dust particles settle on the floor or on other household items, they aren't easily removed by opening windows or using your air purifier. How amazing does it feel to have a freshly deep-cleaned home? Ahhh. Why experience that bliss only here and there? Keep your home tidy, fresh, and clean every day to boost your mood as well as your immune system.

HOUSEHOLD PRODUCTS

Additionally, pay close attention to the household products that you're using. According to Northwest Natural Medicine, the average home has 62 toxic chemicals.[1] Yikes! Natalie was right to start by eliminating any toxic cleaners and products from her home. Anything with toxic ingredients is an endocrine disruptor that will not only disrupt your internal system but will also have a detrimental impact on anyone who comes into your home.

We'll unpack more about makeup, lotion, and skin-care ingredients in part two of this chapter. But, another danger is in any household cleaning products that you may use often. If every single night you're wiping down your kitchen counter with a toxic disinfectant, those toxic chemicals are posing a risk to you and your family. You can begin a cleanout as soon as today by digging through your cleaning cabinet, surveying each list of ingredients on the bottle, and throwing out anything that isn't all-natural or organic.

Here's a list of the most common toxic chemicals found in household products.[2] Look at your air fresheners, countertop sprays, dish soap, polishing agents, and more.

Ammonia is found in polishing agents and glass cleaners and can further irritate asthmatic symptoms or cause chronic bronchitis and asthma. It's especially dangerous for those with already frail lungs.

2-butoxyethanol is found in window and multipurpose cleaners. Not only can it cause a sore throat when inhaled, but it's also linked to narcosis, pulmonary edema, and severe kidney and liver damage.

Chlorine is used in laundry whiteners, toilet bowl cleaners, mildew removers, and some household tap water (we'll talk about water filtration systems later in this chapter). When inhaled or absorbed through the skin, it can disrupt thyroid function and irritate the respiratory system.

Phthalates are commonly found in household products with fragrances. Think about your lavender air fresheners, your lemon-scented dish soap, or even scented toilet papers. Companies don't have to list phthalates on their product labels. So there's no way to know for sure whether your products have it! To be safe and avoid the risk, get rid of products that have a scent. Phthalates are endocrine-disrupting chemicals and can easily be absorbed through the skin.

Quaternary ammonium compounds (quats) are found in household cleaners that say "antibacterial" and in fabric softening liquids and sheets. Quats can cause dermatitis upon skin contact and have also been linked to the development of asthma.

Triclosan is found in many products labeled as "antibacterial": dishwashing detergents, hand soaps, and some mouthwashes and toothpastes. While this seems to be a good feature, there's no real research that backs up why we need this aggressive antibacterial agent. It does more harm than good, as it's a known carcinogen and endocrine disruptor.

Sodium hydroxide is used for oven cleaners and drain openers. As you can expect from its purposes, it is very corrosive. When inhaled, it can cause a sore throat, and when it makes contact with the skin, it can cause severe burns.

Perchloroethylene (perc) is used in many spot removers, carpet cleaners, and dry-cleaning solutions. It's considered to be a neurotoxin and has been linked to dizziness and loss of coordination from extreme exposure.

Thankfully, many companies have created all-natural products as an alternative for these toxic products, many of which are easily accessible at most local stores, such as the Honest

Company, founded by celebrity actress and businesswoman Jessica Alba. One of my favorite things I do for my private clients is an in-home assessment, where we throw out all the old, then restock their home with the most amazing nontoxic items that will leave it feeling fresh and uber clean. I love revamping a home and pantry! It lights me up so much! Netflix, let's get a series . . . yes?

Plastic is also something to look out for in the home. I currently have very young children, and they don't even drink from plastic cups! We use glass mason jar baby bottles. I'm a big proponent of both glass and stainless steel, even with Tupperware. Yes—I admit I like the way the bottles stack nicely and how chic and modern they look in the cabinet (I'm obsessed with simplistic organization!), but really, it's about knowing that I'm actively reducing toxins in my body and my children's bodies simply by making this switch to no plastic. The next section is about heavy metals, and frequently using plastics and Tupperware can contribute to the risk of heavy metal toxicity, not to mention the harmful effects these items have on our planet.

As always, I'll remind you that every little step you take to decrease your environmental stressors will affect your body's Total Toxic Burden. However, you can't expect to throw out one toxic bottle of oven cleaner and be good to go. This requires a holistic look at all irritants, allergens, and pollutants that are infecting your home space, causing the constant production of antibodies within your body on the defense. Each offender affects your sleep and your body's other natural processes, because your body can't work as it's supposed to when it has to fight off irritants and chemicals.

Don't let these recommendations seem overwhelming. Instead, let it be fun! Simplify this and get excited about the new, fresh, clean start that's waiting for you. I'm excited for you to experience it! Go step by step and go for simple. Even the smallest changes to your environmental stressors can make a difference.

HEAVY METAL TOXICITY

Another essential part of assessing environmental factors that cause inflammation is looking at where you may be exposed to heavy metals. The four main heavy metals are mercury, lead, cadmium, and arsenic, but other heavy metals include zinc, nickel, thallium, manganese, cobalt, aluminum, and phosphorus.

Over time, exposure to these heavy metals can cause poisoning when there's too much accumulation in the soft tissues of the body. Symptoms of heavy metal toxicity include headaches, infertility, digestive problems, poor kidney function, memory problems, anxiety, depression, brain fog, tremors, and more—all caused by the inflammation that results from your immune system's response to heavy metals in your body. The symptoms may depend on which heavy metal you have been the most exposed to. For example, lead exposure can lead to lethargy, kidney problems, nausea, diarrhea, headaches, lack of appetite, and abdominal pain, whereas mercury exposure chiefly affects the lungs, brain, and skin.

To know for sure whether or not you have an accumulation of these heavy metals in your body, you can have a heavy metal laboratory test completed through a functional medicine practitioner to check levels of each heavy metal in your body. This will help you know exactly what you're dealing with and what you may need to avoid or reduce in your environment. It's possible you have no idea you have a certain heavy metal built up, and that could be the very thing causing your autoimmune disease or nagging symptoms. This is why I'm such a fan of laboratory testing to identify exactly what's going on inside your body, instead of wasting time and energy trying to guess and check. That said, testing is not always immediately necessary. By reducing any and all exposure to heavy metals, your inflammation may begin to cease on its own without "confirming" what you're dealing with! Start by reducing toxins where you can, then go from there! Your body may just heal itself without any testing when following my anti-inflammatory living recommendations.

How we're exposed to heavy metals

You can be exposed to heavy metals from a number of sources: fertilizers, pesticides, car exhaust, wastewater, paints, and landfills. If you garden frequently and therefore spend a lot of time around fertilizer, you could potentially have high levels of heavy metal toxicity in your body. They can be in the products you use on your body (such as toothpaste, mouthwash, and bar soap) and in your home. Many of today's professions can also entail exposure to these heavy metals: such as being a hairdresser, a laboratory worker, a photographer, a dentist, or a construction worker.[3] The number of heavy metals we're exposed to has increased significantly in the past fifty years because of their use in many of the world's industrial processes and plants. There's simply more in the soil, air, and water than there ever has been before, meaning we have to be on the defensive. Inhaling these toxins is dangerous for our immune systems. I know that this can sound scary, but it's best to be aware! These are stressors that usually go under the radar because we don't think about things around us like the pipes in our home or the products that we use.

Heavy metals can also be present in the food you consume and the water you drink. Crops, such as leafy greens and brown rice, can be high in heavy metals because of the soil, water, and air that they were exposed to, and the fertilizers and growing agents that may have been sprayed on them. You may have heard of mercury poisoning, which could occur from eating too much seafood. This is because the seafood was exposed to mercury in the water, which is why even your favorite seafoods must be consumed in moderation. If you really can't get enough of that shrimp cocktail (we've all been there), note that the higher the quality of the seafood, the smaller the likelihood that it will have as much mercury. Other alerts you may want to know: Mercury can also come from dental fillings in your own mouth. Additionally, processed foods could have heavy metal residue from their processing (another reason to retire all those packaged foods).

The following is a full list of the main heavy metals and where you are most likely to be exposed to them. Again, think of this list as a boost of awareness. This can feel serious and ominous, but awareness is empowerment! The more we can be aware of what's around us, in our food, and in the appliances or products we frequently use or are exposed to, the more we can take control of our Total Toxic Burden.

How do you know which heavy metals you have a higher chance of being exposed to? Do some internet work to find your community or city's public health information. If you're buying or renting a home or apartment, ask some questions about exposure and be hyperconscious in evaluating your products. Thankfully, we're trending away from the use of heavy metals in many manufacturing plants as their danger is becoming more apparent, but it never hurts to be cautious.

Mercury[4] first gets into the air from power-plant emissions.[5] Specifically, in the United States, it's the power plants that burn coal that are the largest source of mercury emissions, and they actually account for 11 percent of all man-made mercury emissions.[6] Other sources can include burning oil, wood, or wastes that contain mercury. Then the airborne mercury eventually settles into bodies of water—specifically, lakes and streams. This is where fish and shellfish may accumulate mercury. The highest levels of methylmercury in fish come from big fish that eat smaller fish.

Lead differs from mercury in that it sticks to soil particles and can sometimes move into groundwater. Fossil fuels, leaded gasoline, lead-based paints, and some types of industrial facilities have contributed to the lead that we can be exposed to. Lead has also been used in products such as cosmetics, batteries, pipes, ceramics, and ammunition. It can enter into drinking water through corroded lead pipes, even if you're in a newer home. "Lead-free" plumbing still can be made of up to 8% lead.[7] Additionally, lead can enter the air from leaded aviation fuel for piston-engine aircraft. Lead in the air is not the real danger; rather, the main concern is lead that has settled from the air into soil, dust, and water.[8]

One common cause of this in soil is when lead-based paint flakes chip off the side of a building or a house and into the soil. Then, children may ingest the lead accidentally after playing in the soil; there's also a risk of lead contamination in vegetables that were grown in the contaminated soil.[9] Lead can settle into dust by the same means: the deterioration of lead-based painted surfaces.

Cadmium is a heavy metal that most often affects the lungs through pulmonary irritation when inhaled. It can also contribute to kidney disease if a buildup of cadmium occurs in the kidneys. According to the Environmental Protection Agency (EPA), cadmium enters the air from the burning of fossil fuels such as coal or oil, and the burning of municipal waste. The EPA also noted that smokers have about *twice as much cadmium* in their bodies as nonsmokers do. For nonsmokers, the risk is from food when phosphate fertilizers were used on farms.[10]

Arsenic, according to the Agency for Toxic Substances and Disease Registry, occurs naturally in soil and minerals. It can enter the air and water from wind-blown dust or runoff. You may ingest arsenic when small amounts are present in your food or water, if you live in an area where there are high levels of arsenic in the rock, or if you work at a job that uses arsenic production such as wood treating, pesticide application, or copper or lead smelting. Ingesting small amounts can cause nausea and vomiting, the sense of "pins and needles" in your hands and feet, and abnormal heart palpitations. Ingesting very high levels can cause death, and breathing in high levels of inorganic arsenic can cause irritated lungs or a sore throat.[11]

Zinc is found in nature and is produced from mining and smelting processes in commercial industries. If you live near a smeltery or a commercial industry, there could be higher levels of zinc in your drinking water, soil, or air. You can ingest or inhale zinc if you breathe air containing zinc, or if small amounts have contaminated food or drinking water through the soil. Now, zinc is also considered an essential nutrient—but in balanced amounts. Too much zinc can cause stomach cramps, nausea, and vomiting, and over time may damage the pancreas and cause nervous system disorders. The Illinois Department of Public Health reported that workers in these smelteries and commercial industries could have "metal fume fever" if they breathe in tremendous amounts of zinc dust and fumes. It's a short illness lasting two days at most, causing chills, excessive sweating, weakness, and fever.[12]

Nickel is also released into the air from the stacks of a power plant. If you live near furnaces that are used to make alloys, trash incinerators, or power plants, you should be aware of potential exposure to nickel. The highest risk is not necessarily by breathing it in, but from food, which is the major source of exposure to nickel as reported by the Agency for Toxic Substances and Disease Registry.[13] You may also be exposed to nickel through the soil and through bath or shower water. It's also possible that you wear jewelry that has nickel, which should be avoided. With all these instances of potential exposure, the amounts are very small—even in food and water.

Thallium is a heavy metal that is used in the manufacturing of electronic devices, switches, and closures. Up until 1972, it was also used as a rat poison, but it is no longer produced in the United States. You can be exposed to thallium through the air, food, and water, but the levels in both air and water are quite low. The greatest risk is in homegrown fruits and vegetables if thallium fell onto the gardens. It can easily be taken up into plants by the roots. Smokers have twice as much thallium in their bodies as nonsmokers do. It most frequently moves to the kidney or the liver, and it can affect your nervous system, lungs, heart, liver, and kidneys.[14]

Manganese, like zinc, is actually necessary for good health when ingested in smaller doses. You could be exposed to high levels from welding factories, or anywhere that steel is made. This puts factory workers at a higher risk. Manganese is present in low levels in water, air, soil, and food, and we are always exposed to some low level of it. The inhalation of manganese in high amounts for workers can affect the nervous system and invoke other behavioral changes.

Cobalt enters the environment from nickel and copper mining and from burning coal and oil. It is considered to be widely distributed throughout the environment, and we are exposed to it mainly through food and drinking water. This can be avoided by thoroughly cleaning garden vegetables. High amounts of cobalt inhalation can cause asthma, pneumonia, and wheezing, and ingesting high amounts of cobalt can lead to thyroid damage, vomiting, vision problems, dermatitis, and even death.

Aluminum is actually the most abundant metal from the earth's crust, and is used to make planes, roofing, siding, foil, pots, pans, and beverage cans. A powdered version is also used for explosives and fireworks, and it may be found in food additives, antiperspirants, cosmetics, and antacids. You are most likely to be exposed to aluminum through food: namely, baking powder, flour, and coloring agents. According to the Agency for Toxic Substances and Disease Registry, the average adult in the US eats about 7–9 mg of aluminum per day in their food. It is far less commonly found in the air or the water. Though studies have been done, it is inconclusive if high levels of aluminum can lead to Alzheimer's disease. Bone, brain, and kidney disease have also been thought to be linked to high amounts of aluminum. The best way to avoid exposure to aluminum is to avoid processed foods whenever you can, and to consider using pots made from stainless steel or glass instead of aluminum.[15] You could also try parchment paper instead of aluminum foil when baking!

Phosphorus is used to manufacture smoke bombs, explosives, pyrotechnics, artificial fertilizers, and rodenticides—yeah. You know where this is heading! White phosphorus particularly is extremely toxic to humans. The main risk of being exposed is for those who work in the munitions industries. It can cause gastrointestinal distress, vomiting, and liver, respiratory, and kidney effects. If it comes in contact with your skin, it can cause severe burns.[16]

OXIDATIVE FREE RADICALS

If the buildup of heavy metals occurs in the body, it leads to the production of oxidative free radicals. Oxidative stress is what we want to avoid, which is why foods high in *anti*oxidants are considered so important, since antioxidants help to mitigate the effect of free radicals. In short, free radicals are the result of what happens when oxygen molecules become stressed and split up into two single atoms. Now their electrons are unpaired, so the atoms are "free radicals" (or atoms without a paired electron), which then search high and low throughout the body for an electron to pair with. In the process, this can cause a lot of damage. It's simply another form of an imbalance. Oxidative stress leads to inflammation, and can cause issues such as diabetes, cancer, high blood sugar, aging, high blood pressure, and really any symptom at all.

This oxidative stress is just an addition to the other symptoms that result from heavy metal buildup. Heavy metals are one of the body's biggest inflammatory stressors. While we can't always protect ourselves from them, we can make choices that lower our degree of exposure, such as small lifestyle changes as outlined in this book.

PURIFYING YOUR WATER

Water intake is so important—not only to flush out the body and naturally hydrate you but also for your skin! Skin is the largest organ of the body, and its cells—just like all our cells—are composed mainly of water. When dehydrated, your skin shows it. It may appear cracked, dry, or irritated if it hasn't been adequately hydrated. This doesn't mean you should apply more moisturizer—rather, drink a few more glasses of water to aid in the hydration! According to the University of Wisconsin, Madison, water actually reaches all the organs *before* it reaches the skin.[17] So you could be adequately hydrating everything *except* for your skin.

Water should be something you have on hand, all day. It's advised to drink eight glasses of eight ounces of water every day—at *least*. This is a baseline habit! The hardest part can be remembering to keep drinking, so try to keep a water bottle with you throughout the day—at your desk or wherever you spend the most time. You can also use an app that reminds you to drink water—there are plenty available in your phone's app store! Some people believe they need to drink a gallon of water every single day, but I advise against this unless it's happening as a one-time thing because you're doing a detox week or a water fast. You should drink more than eight glasses of eight ounces of water in a day if you're physically active and sweating a lot, if you're pregnant, or if you're breastfeeding—but even then, not a gallon long-term for most people.

Additionally, adding lemons to the water can make it a bit tastier to drink, and lemon water has its own added benefits. I always start the morning with a glass of lemon water because it's a great reset for the digestive system and is infinitely hydrating. Lemon juice also serves as an antioxidant, which can defend against oxidative stress in your body. Squeeze a fresh lemon half into your big glass of water, then drop the rest of the lemon in. It tastes great, and you'll feel even greater!

Another great antioxidant to add to water is a handful of frozen berries. If you throw a few frozen blueberries and raspberries into your water bottle, it will infuse the water with the antioxidants from the fruit. That said, remember we're limiting fruit, aside from a few berries in the morning, because of all the natural sugar, so let the berry-infused water be a sweet treat sometimes.

I also love using matcha tea powder in my water. I first heat the water, then whisk in the matcha tea powder. It is chock-full of antioxidants—in fact, it's said to have 137 times as many antioxidants as green tea does! And it has nearly 17 times as many antioxidants as blueberries do.[18] I'll also do a matcha latte as a coffee alternative to start my morning off with a super anti-inflammatory beverage, made by mixing the matcha tea powder in with warm nut milk.

Last, but definitely not least, one of the best things you can do to boost your system from the inside out is to get a good night's sleep!

Another one of my staple recommendations is to invest in a high-quality water filtration system! My plan for clients always includes the introduction of a high-quality water filter, because about 30% of plumbing infrastructure in the US contains lead piping, lead service lines, or lead plumbing components, which can easily make its way into your water.[19] Even if you think the water in your home is OK, you're worth the extra step to make sure it's purified water. A report by the Natural Resources Defense Council (NRDC) found a number of other water contaminants across the nation's tap-water supply, and these were contaminants with potentially carcinogenic ramifications. Some pathogens found in the tap water, such as cryptosporidium or giardia, can lead to digestive distress like diarrhea and nausea. According to the NRDC's analysis, in 2015 alone "there were more than 80,000 reported violations of the Safe Drinking Water Act by community water systems. Nearly 77 million people were served by more than 18,000 of these systems with violations in 2015."[20]

So, each time you're drinking from a sink or a drinking fountain, or you're drinking any type of poorly filtered water, you are possibly introducing bacteria, heavy metals, traces of pharmaceutical medications, and so much more into your body. The same goes for the ice you add into your smoothies or drinks if you aren't using properly filtered water to make the ice. These bacteria and toxins could also be in the showers and baths you take if you aren't doing the extra steps to filter that water as well. The water you submerge yourself in when you're taking a bath or rinse under when you're taking a shower actually goes into your body! It's just as important as the water that you consume internally.

I know—it's scary! Especially because water transports everything in your body—it comes in contact with your cells, lubricates your connective tissue, and performs important functions like regulating temperature and transferring heat. Since the skin is the largest organ of our body, and our body is made up of mostly water, it's essential to take this seriously.

The best line of defense we can use is a water filtration system—and I'm sorry, but if you just have one of those standard refrigerator water filters, it's not enough. It needs to be a high-quality system that thoroughly filters the water—otherwise it won't work and your water will still have toxins. As of the time writing this book, some great brands to check into are Home Master, Aquasana, and Berkey for top water filtration systems. You can head to maggieberghoff.com for any updated recommendations!

My top recommendation for filter systems is to get an under-sink water filter. It's installed under your kitchen sink and there's a separate spout at your sink solely for the super-clean water. Since the filter is under the sink, you don't even have to think about it and you'll have an abundance of great water (no filling up a tank every day). Just turn on your water when washing your fruits and vegetables or filling up your water bottle for the day, and the filter will eliminate any and all heavy metals, pollutants, pharmaceuticals, and chemicals. If you live in an apartment or you're traveling and can't go through the process of installing an under-sink water filter, there are many great travel or temporary water filters, too, like the Berkey I recommended. With these, you can keep a filter on your countertop and simply add water to it. It will filter for you, so the water that comes out of it is clean. Just make sure the brand of the filter you choose is trusted and credible, and that the filters specifically eliminate all of the concerns. You may notice that your water tastes better as a result of using filters, too! I love the security of knowing the water that I'm drinking and that my family is drinking (and even bathing or showering in) is the best and cleanest water.

You can even do some visualization with this! Every time you fill your cup, think of how pure and amazing your water is. Every time you take a sip, imagine that water going throughout your body healing it. Even say in your mind a little message or prayer as that water goes in: "Please go throughout my body . . . every organ . . . every system . . . and please please heal me." Try it out!

Wrapping up, a great water filter will clear out any and all heavy metals from your tap water: lead, nickel, cadmium, mercury, and chromium, in addition to any other contaminants that may have entered the water supply, such as pesticides, toxins, and bacteria. Having a water filter is mandatory.

RED-LIGHT THERAPY

It's not often talked about, but another one of the main recommendations for you is to use red-light therapy. Red-light therapy has been shown to reduce inflammation and other aches and pains within your body. This is done through using red-light therapy devices, and you can purchase them for use in the comfort of your home! Red-light therapy increases the amount of energy that our cells have. In other words, it makes the cells "supercharged"—so that they can give us the energy that we need for healing. It's really quite cool—like "food" for our cells via light! Our cells are already custom-made to do everything in their power to help reduce inflammation and take care of our bodies. But when they're stressed out due to our Total Toxic Burden being high, they can use all the help that they can get.

Red-light therapy regenerates the cells. Think of it as a bolt of the highest-quality delicious espresso to the cells that are the most tired. Instant gratification. The red light creates a chemical reaction in the cell's mitochondria, which can reduce oxidative stress and create a better oxidative environment for your cells. And . . . voila! Your cells once again have the energy to do their best work! As the cells are supercharged, we too become a bit invincible! I'm all in the business of thriving—and red-light therapy helps you do just that. You know that I don't believe it's normal to have constant digestive problems, PMS, fatigue, sleep issues, anxiety, or depression—sure, it's common, but if we can supercharge our cells and step into our most vibrant health, we can truly feel great all of the time.

Many studies have been completed on red-light therapy's rejuvenation powers. For joint inflammation, one notable 2018 study in Brazil showed decreased cytokine levels and increased immune cell populations after red-light therapy was given. Another study found that morning stiffness was delayed by an average of 27.5 minutes because of red-light therapy. It can also be helpful with producing melatonin and ensuring a more restful night's sleep. Another study backed up the claim on more restful sleep and also showed great success among individuals with sleep disorders. These powerful benefits comprise many of the reasons why I personally use red-light therapy and recommend it so consistently to my clients, and I encourage you to try it, too. It's also great for healing post injury or surgery. Give your cells a helping hand in the right direction so that they can help you heal with red-light therapy.

LIGHT

Going back to the days before the introduction of the light bulb (crazy to think there was a time like that!), humans naturally rose with the sunrise, and when after sunset it was dimmed and dark, they fell asleep in darkness. Our natural circadian rhythms, the biological clock of the body, correspond with the natural rise and fall of the sun to allow our body to function at its best. However, due to artificial light, blue light from our computer and phone screens all day and into the night, waking up in the wee hours of the morning before the sun comes up, and sleeping with city lights coming in through our windows, our circadian rhythm is impacted negatively. And when our circadian rhythm is "off," everything is off. This has led to many less-than-ideal symptoms in the majority of humans. One is waking up tired and groggy, even if you slept your normal eight hours the night before. Or, tossing and turning at night not able to fall asleep or stay asleep.

Another issue related to sleep is waking up in the middle of the night for "no reason." A circadian rhythm disruption can also lead to afternoon slumps and feeling tired, hungry, or groggy in the midafternoon. Unrelated to sleep and energy, circadian rhythm disturbance can also contribute to weight complications and unhealthy body composition, cravings, anxiety and depression, and so much more. How frustrating!

Our natural circadian rhythms happen over a 24-hour period (if we break down the Latin term circadian into "circa" and "diem," it means "around one day") and determine many of the cycles that our body is responsible for: beyond sleeping, that includes appetite, digestion, and more. If you've ever flown around the world and experienced extreme jet lag, that was the result of a clash between your body's circadian rhythm and the time zone of the new city you arrived in. In addition to symptoms like total exhaustion during the day and being wide awake and starving at 4:00 a.m., you may also have felt sick because of the disruption of your circadian rhythm. This is why some people can't stand waking up before the sunrise for an early morning flight, for example. If it makes your whole body feel "ick," the same is also true when you stay up too late past dark staring into the blue light of a laptop, TV, or cell phone!

If you really want to get well and feel your best, light is definitely something we need to look at in your environment. Let's get into some quick tips right now so you can start implementing them today.

Let's start with the very beginning of your day. You just woke up—what next? First, if at all possible, I want you to wake up *only if* the sun is rising or is already up . . . not when it's still dark outside. You can find out around what time the sun rises in your area, then set your alarm accordingly. Hopefully, over time, your body will naturally wake up at that time without the alarm, as that's what a properly set circadian rhythm and biological clock will do. I know you have that friend, partner, or family member who wakes up and goes to sleep at the same times every day and night without an alarm clock and with ease. It seems like a superpower . . . but that's possible for you, too! You have the same internal clock, and it's ready to be synchronized with the sun. There's something pretty cool about that if you ask me.

Next, step out of your bed with intention and excitement to begin the day. Be grateful and positive the moment those eyes blink open! Open the door that leads you outside, step out into the crisp morning air, look up to that rising sun, and breathe. Getting outside first thing in the morning is so helpful. It activates little clock genes on our skin and in our eyes (so don't put on those sunglasses quite yet!) and starts the energy-making cells in our body. It tells our biological clock that yes, indeed, it is morning and time to start the day! Plus, it's so great to get into nature, breathe fresh air, and expose your skin to sunlight (in the right doses of course).

Go about your morning routine after you've taken these important steps.

Getting natural light in the afternoon is the next most important step in setting your circadian rhythm. If you have an office job and have to stay inside all day, try to walk outside briefly on your lunch break for even five to ten minutes. I promise it will do you wonders to step into the fresh air, get out of your routine for a moment, take some slow breaths through your nose, let your skin feel the sun's rays. From a mental and biochemical standpoint, it's a necessity.

When I walk outside, I sometimes go barefoot in order to ground my body. I soak in the sunshine in order to allow my body to synthesize vitamin D, which in fact isn't a vitamin at all. It's actually a hormone that's essential for immunity and for many functions within the body. Research has found that immune cells in autoimmune diseases are responsive to the ameliorative effects of vitamin D, which may assist in auto-immune diseases.[21] I also take a few, grounding, deep breaths through my nose. These actions each seem so small and so simple, but the practices make a major and wonderful differ-ence to the body's ability to stay in sync.

Next up is evening light! Get outside again while the sun is setting—trust me. The rays from the setting sun will actually activate the sleep hormone melatonin in your body, which helps you get prime sleep. This is an essential factor for anyone trying to achieve health and wellness goals!

Once back inside, make sure that beautiful, setting sun evening light isn't disturbed by all your bright inside lights. There are a few ways to help aid this transition. One, you can get light bulbs that change from normal "day light" to an amber or darker yellow tint for evening time. You can also simply add an amber- or red-tinted light bulb to a few lamps in each room and designate them to turn on in the evening. You can also find great amber- or red-tinted night-lights that we love to use for hallways and bathrooms, to be sure we don't ruin our circadian rhythm with bright lights in those areas. This is especially important for me personally, as I have young kids and do need to wake up throughout the night to help the toddler go back to sleep after a dream, to tend to the baby, or to feed the newborn. I had three babies in three years at the time of writing this book, so making sure I do everything I can to keep my circadian rhythm in check is essential! It's what makes all the difference in the efficacy of my sleep and my energy for the day.

Now that our light bulbs are in check for the evening and nighttime, let's focus on the light from our devices! I want you to red-tint your computer and phone screens in the evening. There's usually an app with an automatic timer available that will change this for you, so you never have to even think about it. Go into your phone settings and check for "night mode." For your computer, at the time of this writing, there's a free download called "f.lux" that you can put on your computer to make it red-tinted in the evening! Both are awesome game changers—free and effective.

BLUE LIGHT AND ITS NEGATIVE IMPACTS

The reason I mention your phone and computer light is due to what's called *blue light*. It's called blue light in reference to the UV scale; blue has the shortest wavelength and the highest amount of energy. Sunlight has blue light—but it also has red, orange, yellow, and green light. LED and fluorescent lights also have blue light, as does the glow of your phone or laptop.

When observed by your eye's optic nerve, this blue light contributes to feelings of alertness and increased focus, and can increase your heart rate, too. Of course, these man-made instances of blue light have only a fraction of the sun's blue light, but it still has an impact. When we're on our phones, computers, or watching TV beyond when the sun sets, we're continuously exposed to blue light, which confuses our body's circadian rhythm. The same is true when we have artificial lights on in our house. Too much exposure to artificial light past the time of sunset can lead the circadian rhythm to either lengthen or shorten from its 24-hour period.

That type of disturbance is certain to cause an imbalance within the circadian rhythm, which can negatively impact the body's ability to fall asleep and stay asleep. According to research,[22] "Rather recently, the availability of artificial light has substantially changed the light environment, especially during evening and night hours. This may increase the risk of developing circadian rhythm sleep-wake disorders (CRSWD). . . . While the exact relationship between the availability of artificial light and CRSWD remains to be established, nocturnal light has been shown to alter circadian rhythms and sleep in humans."

Your body takes cues from the light it's exposed to. Your body doesn't know that it's time to go to sleep if it's exposed to bright lights until the very moment you finish brushing your teeth and hop into bed. That's like standing out in the sun and expecting to signal to every cell in your body that it's bedtime! When you finally put your phone down or close your laptop and close your eyes, you're still energized and alert from exposure to the blue light. This creates insomnia—or, if you do fall right to sleep, you may not have as deep and restful of sleep, so you're likely to wake up still tired.

Research from *Endocrine Reviews* found that "although outdoor light levels do not always reflect retinal light exposure, about 75% of the world's population is exposed to artificial light at night, and it has been estimated that individuals in modern societies commonly experience light intensity levels over *twice as high* between sunset and sleep compared to exposure to only natural light."[23] No wonder everything is falling out of sync! At night, we're close to the glow of our phones, computers, and TVs, and as a result can be even more alert than during the day, when exposed to natural sunlight. If you find that you are more energized and work better at night, and therefore call yourself a "night owl," it may just be because you're more exposed to blue light at night and your body is confused. But although being a "night owl" may be something you enjoy because you get a lot of work done or have more alone time, it's disrupting your circadian rhythm, which can lead to unwanted symptoms and conditions long-term, so don't make it a habit.

The effects of blue light on circadian rhythms go beyond the disruptive bouts of insomnia. A study at Harvard[24] found that those who extended their circadian rhythms by staying up later (thanks to the effect of blue light) experienced a rise in blood sugar—a substantial enough rise to make them prediabetic. Further, their leptin levels decreased. Leptin is the hormone that helps the body determine that it's full and has had enough to eat. Based on this study, it's likely that the disruption of our circadian rhythms from artificial light increases the risk of diabetes and obesity.

The *Endocrine Review* went on to report that "disrupted sleep, for example, promotes increased energy intake, reduced energy expenditure, and insulin resistance in many individuals, consequences that may be compounded by an increased propensity to make less healthy dietary choices."

A lack of sleep can also lead to weight gain. A study by the *Proceedings of the National Academy of Sciences* included 16 adults in a 15-day inpatient study with five days of insufficient sleep.[25] Their findings suggested that "increased food intake during insufficient sleep is a physiological adaptation to provide energy needed to sustain additional wakefulness; yet when food is easily accessible, intake surpasses that needed." Additionally, their findings demonstrated "physiological and behavioral mechanisms by which insufficient sleep may contribute to overweight and obesity."

While it may be difficult to eliminate blue-light influences fully past sundown—especially in the depths of winter, when the sun sets before dinnertime, or if you live in the city where streetlights are beaming into your window—being cognizant of your exposure to blue light is critical. It's not always about being perfect, it's simply about making a few switches to help improve your own environment where you can! The iPhone recently introduced a feature that can dim the typical blue light of the phone to yellow light via "nighttime mode." There's also an app available that works as a "blue-light filter," so you can turn it on past sunset when you're getting ready for bed. Or, buy a pair of blue-light glasses if you have no choice but to finish up some work or answer some emails before bed.

Scheduling a specific time for turning off technology every night is a great first step to getting your circadian rhythm back to its natural sync. Turn off phones, laptops, and televisions, and instead read, stretch, or meditate in the hour before bed. Keep all technology out of sight and out of mind! This will give your body the time and environment it needs to prepare for sleep, so you fall asleep faster and stay asleep longer.

I always say that the body knows what to do to heal itself. But when it's exposed to stressors and disruptions that cause internal imbalances, it's hard for it to maintain the homeostasis it needs to function properly. Blue light in excess, and at the wrong times, is indeed a stressor. The body needs its valuable sleep in order to heal, and your body needs to be in sync with its natural rhythm to perform its natural processes.

Trying to lose weight, heal autoimmune disease, look younger, have more energy, and get rid of nagging symptoms? Get your light right.

ELECTROMAGNETIC FIELDS (EMFS)

EMFs, or electromagnetic fields, are something that I must mention when we're talking about environmental stressors. It's definitely a topic that we need to consider more and more, as the world and its technology advances. I'm a big fan of technology—I use it all the time and love the luxury and convenience it offers. I don't want you to be afraid of it or attempt to live in isolation without any modern technological devices in your home. However, I want to talk about what we can do to live in a modern world and enjoy a modern lifestyle while still combating some of the harmful effects of EMFs in a way that's simple and realistic. EMF exposure can relate to either the area where you live (which may have a higher electromagnetic charge) or simply exposure to appliances like our microwaves, cell phones, and Wi-Fi routers. Excess exposure to this type of radiation is thought to cause damage to cells and DNA. The problem is that each individual device that emits EMFs—our cell phones, the security at the airport, our laptops, Bluetooth, etc.—may be OK on its own due to the "low levels" and "safe levels" marketers claim that they have. However, the truth of the matter is that we *aren't* exposed to "low/safe" levels. We are exposed to endless EMFs all day, every day, in just about everything nowadays! And since we're exposed to all of them at once, those so-called low levels add up now to chronically high levels of EMF onto our body each and every day. Make sense? It's the combination effect.

One recommendation is to spend as much time with the earth as possible—hear me out! This process called "earthing," which is being barefoot outdoors, reduces free radicals and inflammation from our toxic environments. It can really help to rebalance and recalibrate our body.

The more time you can spend in nature barefoot, the better. I enjoy doing a bit of visualization just as I do when I eat a nutrient-packed meal. I close my eyes, feel the grass beneath the soles of my feet and between my toes, and imagine the earth's grounding, rooting energy coming up through the center of my feet. I feel my connection to the world around me and meditate on the stability of it for just a few minutes. I love this little ritual! And—even better—it can work for decreasing inflammation in the body.

Gaetan Chevalier, Gregory Melvin, and Tiffany Barsotti conducted a study with forty middle-aged volunteers to understand the impact of grounding on inflammation and circulation.[26] They split the volunteers into two groups—the test group and the control group—and had the test group sit in recliner chairs with grounding mats and pillows. They used thermal imaging to determine whether or not there was an increase in facial circulation.

As stated in their findings, "Thermal imaging showed clearly improved circulation of fluids (including blood) throughout the torso, which in turn translates into enhanced delivery of blood to the head and improved blood circulation in the face as well. The results of this innovative study demonstrate that even one-hour contact with the Earth appears to promote significantly autonomic nervous system control of body fluids and peripheral blood flow that may improve blood circulation in the torso and face, facial tissue repair, skin health and vitality and optimize facial appearance."

The more time you can spend outside, barefoot in the grass, the better for your body's overall circulation. It's a great trick to help you mitigate the toxic stressors that you're often exposed to. One of my favorite tips for my clients who are frequent travelers is to ground barefoot outside in the grass as soon as they are able to after their flight lands. This technique is such a game changer in resetting the body right away for a healthy and energetic trip, or to rebound when you get home from traveling. It's like checking in with the earth and your body saying, "Hey, we need to recalibrate quickly. Thanks!" We really do have that level of communication between our bodies and our environments.

Another thing we can do to reduce our EMF exposure is to reduce the number of devices we're using. Do you really need to track your steps with a Bluetooth device strapped on your wrist all day? Do you even really use it? Look at the electronics you are using and ensure that you actually care enough about them to allow the exposure. As with everything, there's a cost-and-benefit analysis. If you use technology that tracks your sleep, activity, and body temperature, and this makes you feel more empowered and in control of your body and your health, then it's probably worth the minimal amount of EMF exposure. But if you are wearing technology or keeping your phone near you all the time just to stay up-to-date on your latest social media notifications, maybe create some boundaries for both your mental health and your overall health.

In addition, you can set up your office in a way that decreases EMFs by wiring in your computers instead of relying on Wi-Fi all day. Another idea would be to distance yourself from your devices. Get that cell phone off your body. Keep it an arm's length away from you at minimum. Don't sleep with it by your head at night, don't keep it in your pocket all day, and don't constantly scroll aimlessly for hours on end. I know . . . it's habitual! The cycle can be hard to break, but there are now great resources even within our technology that will sound off a timer if we've been on for too long. Take control of your life by setting clear limitations, so you can be reminded if you've gone above and beyond your time limit on the phone. Sometimes just that little nudge of "Remember your commitment to being present away from technology?" can be enough to pull you back into productivity. Detoxing and taking a break from all technology can also be so beneficial from time to time, even if it's just for one hour of your day. Turn off your phone (or at least put it in airplane mode), close that computer, and turn off the bright lights.

PART TWO: OPTIMIZING YOUR SKIN'S ANTI-INFLAMMATORY BARRIER

We talked extensively about what you're ingesting (through real, whole foods and properly filtered water) and breathing (purified air), but what you put on your skin is of equal importance. What you apply on your skin and on your face is absorbed into your system. I always like to tell people, "If you wouldn't eat your lotion, don't put it on your skin." It sounds gross to imagine eating a big spoonful of lotion like it's yogurt, but if it's on your body, it will *enter* your body just like what you ingest does! That's a serious consideration.

So, an important component of decreasing environmental stressors is talking about skin care—not necessarily a "skin-care routine" but my best practices for taking care of my skin; avoiding toxic and harmful ingredients in makeup, skin care, and lotion; lymphatic drainage; and other tips that can reduce swelling.

INGREDIENTS TO AVOID

First and foremost, we must get rid of any toxic ingredients that you may be putting on your body without knowing it! For your makeup, skin care, and lotion, look carefully at the ingredient labels to make sure you aren't purchasing anything with parabens, alcohol, formaldehyde, phthalates, sodium lauryl sulfate, or added fragrances. Also evaluate the products you currently have, and throw out anything with the ingredients listed below! During my own health crisis, I was wearing a heavily fragrant (and so, a heavily *toxic*) lotion every single day! I look back and totally gawk at that choice, now that I know how much it was stressing out my body. Luckily, many all-natural makeup, lotion, and skin-care brands have been founded in recent years, so you have an abundant array to pick from. A good rule of thumb is that the all-natural products will have only a few main ingredients, and they'll be recognizable or you'll know what they are.

To help you out, I've listed here the top offending ingredients that are commonly found in beauty products that I'd love for you to avoid.[27] As with all of these "restrictive" lists, the intention is to empower and to educate!

Ingredients to Avoid in Beauty Products[28]

Benzalkonium chloride can cause severe irritation in the skin, eyes, and respiratory system. It's more commonly found in sunscreen and moisturizers.

Butylated hydroxy anisole and **butylated hydroxytoluene** are both synthetic antioxidants used to extend the shelf lives of lipsticks and diaper creams. They may cause liver damage and are also endocrine disruptors.

Coal-tar hair dyes are by-products of coal processing. They are commonly found in hair dye and shampoo and contain known carcinogens.

Ethylenediaminetetraacetic acid (EDTA) is found in hair color and moisturizers and is considered to likely be toxic to organs.

Formaldehyde is a common preservative for cosmetics. It's linked to asthma, neurotoxicity, and developmental toxicity. It can be found in shampoo, bubble-bath products, and body wash.

Hydroquinone is used in skin-lightening creams but can inhibit melanin production and has been linked to cancer, skin irritation, and organ toxicity.

Methylisothiazolinone and **methylchloroisothiazolinone** are chemical preservatives found in shampoo, conditioner, and body wash that can cause skin allergies or reaction upon contact.

Oxybenzone is commonly found in sunscreen or SPF moisturizers but can irritate the skin and can also act as an endocrine disruptor.

Parabens (such as methyl-, isobutyl-, propyl-, and others) are preservatives used to prevent the growth of bacteria and mold in shampoo, body wash, body lotion, foundation, and facial cleanser. Parabens are considered endocrine disruptors.

Phthalates (DBP, DEHP, DEP, and others) are chemicals that help fragrances stick to the skin and can also help to make products stick to the body. They are often used in synthetic fragrances, hairspray, nail polish, and plastic materials. They are endocrine disruptors and may cause birth defects.

Polyethylene glycols (PEGs) are in sunscreens, creams, and shampoos. Due to their manufacturing process, they may have been contaminated with carcinogenic chemicals.

Retinyl palmitate (vitamin A palmitate) is a common ingredient in some retinol creams. It has been thought to contribute to some health consequences such as lesions and photosensitization.

Sodium lauryl sulfate and **sodium laureth sulfate** are commonly found in body wash, shampoo, and bubble-bath products. They are usually contaminated with 1,4-dioxane.

Synthetic flavors or fragrances can contain up to three thousand chemical ingredients, but fragrance formulas are produced under the federal law for "trade secrets." All types of cosmetics with synthetic flavors and fragrances should be subject to scrutiny and avoided.

Toluene is a petrochemical solvent found in nail polish that can cause birth defects and be toxic to the immune system.

Triclosan and **triclocarban** are found in toothpaste, liquid soap, and soap bars, and can harm reproductive systems.[29]

All of these environmental stressors—polluted water, allergens and irritants in the air, heavy metals, improper light—are important in achieving, preventing, and maintaining optimal health and vitality. It's the combination of these small changes that can help the body start to heal, helping any and all types of inflammation.

Choose just one or two areas to write down from this chapter to focus on improving in your life this week. Share with me what you choose on social media! Tag me so I'm sure to see it—I really want to know, and it will help keep you accountable. Did you buy some amber night-lights for the bedroom, bathroom? Did you just put a time-limit on your phone because you can't stop scrolling Instagram? Or, maybe you are choosing to have your home deep-cleaned this week to get rid of dust and allergens (with nontoxic cleaning products as a bonus . . . what a treat!). Whatever it is, however small, it matters, and I'm so proud of you for taking action. These little steps are actually HUGE steps because of how they will combine to help you live your healthiest and most vibrant life.

11

SUPERCHARGE YOUR IMMUNE SYSTEM

Now, we can't have an entire book about inflammation without discussing the immune system. In fact, inflammation is one of the soldiers deployed by the immune system to keep your body safe and to fight against any type of infection or virus. We've talked a lot about best practices for keeping our Total Toxic Burden down and managed so that our bodies are stronger and less prone to illness. What we're doing by reducing the number of offenders and stressors is supercharging our immune system so it can protect us even better. Do you want a supercharged immune system? Keep reading.

I like to think of the immune system as an invincible army within the body that works day and night to handle any of the stressors that come our way. And, in today's world especially, those stressors can be frequent and consistent. They can span from our toddler sneezing after getting home from preschool to pressing an elevator button that hasn't been sanitized in months to an old tomato that accidentally ended up in our salad. Here's the thing, though: there's no way to protect ourselves against all these potential offenders, even if we decided to wear hazmat suits every time we left the house. That said, it's not my intention to scare you. The immune system doesn't *expect* that we stay away from every potential offender. In fact, the immune system's entire responsibility is as the "cleanup crew" for when we inevitably meet some of these germs in our environment. Protecting us is exactly what it was meant and built to do—and it does a great job of it, especially when we take measures to supercharge it. When it doesn't turn out so great for us is when our immune systems are compromised and not strong like they should be.

WHAT DOES THE IMMUNE SYSTEM DO?

Let's meet some of the "behind-the-scenes" soldiers that work within the immune system to keep us safe. You may have learned about white blood cells, or leukocytes. Think of these as the white knights of your body. A whole crew of leukocytes is constantly swimming throughout all the blood vessels in your body, looking for any toxins, waste, or anything that isn't supposed to be there. Then, they kindly but firmly escort these toxins off the premises once they have been located.

Once a toxin has been identified, the leukocytes rush to rid your body of the waste in only minutes. It's truly amazing! That means that while you're out for a stroll with friends or making dinner and minding your own business, your leukocytes are hard at work to make sure you're safe and that all threats have been removed. Take a moment to revel in that, and even feel it in your body. Imagine this army that has worked tirelessly for your health and well-being all of your life.

This army is multitalented, too. Because antigens that bring on strep throat are quite different from the antigens present when you're battling food poisoning, every leukocyte (or "soldier") has a different specialty.

There's a type of leukocyte called a phagocyte, and when it detects an antigen, it engulfs it. Once it does so, it's able to signal and transmit information on the antigen to the rest of the leukocytes in the body. So, not only is your immune system composed of leukocytes that work tirelessly for your defense, but they're basically telepathic, too!

With this information, the T cells search for infected cells and get to work taking care of the situation. And B cells and helper T cells begin to produce antibodies, which will defend your body against any potential further infection. Think of it this way: imagine that a coworker gets sick and you accidentally pick up her pen. The "sickness" of whatever your coworker has gets into your body, and this entire defense process begins. The leukocytes spring into action and the phagocytes engulf the antigens. The danger is gone! Well, imagine that the next day you go back to work, and another one of your coworkers also feels herself coming down with something because of the originally sick coworker. The presence of antibodies will help your body fight against any additional exposure in a less taxing and more efficient way, because the leukocytes already know what to look out for. When your immune system is not fully strengthened, however, the opposite happens—you get that sickness from said coworker.

Ever since you were born, your immune system has become even smarter and stronger with every antigen that it's defended you from. It will never stop learning and growing to protect you. But, just like us when we're worn out, the immune system needs rest and support to do its best work. If the immune system is constantly in overdrive because a body's Total Toxic Burden is through the roof, it's going to work less efficiently and over-tire, simply because it's working constantly to defend against the many stressors the body is exposed to.

These stressors don't just mean bacteria or anything that can get us sick. The immune system also springs into action if we spray a fragrant perfume on our wrists, when we walk outside into smog, when we walk past a pesticide-sprayed weed on our neighbor's lawn, or when we eat too many processed, chemical-laden foods. These are all viable stressors. While many of them are unavoidable (such as the air quality outside or being exposed to cleaning chemicals in a public restroom), there are many stressors that *are* avoidable. The more you can keep your Total Toxic Burden down by reducing the stressors, the stronger your immune system will be. The more we can decrease inflammation, the stronger your immune system will be.

A strong immune system goes beyond protecting us from sickness. It can protect us from infection, help us heal more quickly after surgery or a traumatic event, support a healthy pregnancy, and keep us feeling our best even when we're worn down from frequent traveling or long nights at the office. We just have to help the immune system in the same way it's helping us.

IMMUNITY AND FOOD

Eat to fuel your body. Eat to feel amazing. Eat to thrive.

If your body has all the nutrients it needs, you're going to have a far better outcome when you're exposed to bacteria, viruses, parasites, and toxins.

Now, I've shared with you that I don't believe in total restriction. However, some of my clients find it helpful to know the foods and drinks that can hurt their immune systems. I'm not telling you to totally nix these and never look back, but rather to be aware. Next time you feel like your throat is getting sore or you're coming down with something—or, you're about to have a long day of traveling and you know you always feel worn down and vulnerable to sickness when you do—maybe hold off on some of these immune-system foes. Decreasing inflammatory foods will surely boost your body's ability to defend you when it's under attack.

Alcohol. Again, I love a good cocktail as much as the next gal, but when focusing on boosting the immune system, alcohol is not your friend. Opt for organic, sugar-free wine if you're going to enjoy a drink. My favorite brand is called Dry Farm Wines. All my favorite brands and companies are always linked on my website store, so head there for other recommendations!

Anything high in sugar content. It's going to be challenging for your hard-working leukocyte soldiers to be on patrol for antigens if they keep getting bogged down by sugar in your bloodstream! There are plenty of other ways to satisfy your sweet tooth while your body recovers, with foods that help your immune system. Try a dark chocolate bar or a handful of berries! If nothing else, at least swap to natural sugars, like honey.

Processed foods. While, sometimes, nothing sounds better than lying on the couch with a bag of potato chips when you're feeling run-down, try to stay away from any of the processed foods. These chemicals work as stressors to the body, giving the leukocytes extra work, which can distract them or spread them thin. It will definitely tank your immune system due to the inflammation hit you'll be getting.

Consuming these foods or drinks is like when you're already on a tight deadline and a client or your boss throws in another big project on top of it. Be the cool boss and send in the immune-boosting snacks instead to give you a boost!

EPSOM SALT BATHS

One of my favorite anti-inflammatory practices is to take a nice, soothing, Epsom salt bath! I run warm water, then add a few cups of Epsom salts. Make sure to check the ingredient labels on your Epsom salt packages, or anything you're going to put in your bath (including bath bombs or bubble-bath ingredients). Why would you want to soak in toxic chemicals? Make sure the ingredients are strictly Epsom salts or magnesium salts. Add a few drops of essential oils to make it extra dreamy. I recommend getting lavender for deep relaxation, and then a few premade blends, such as an "Immune Boosting" blend. I make my baths super relaxing—I turn on some music, listen to a podcast, read a book, or put my laptop on a stool next to the bathtub to watch a show—a rare occurrence for me!

You can take an Epsom salt bath every single day if you want, but I definitely recommend at least once a week and, ideally, two to three times per week! All you need is thirty minutes to set aside for this soak. I think you'll come to look forward to it, as it truly is so relaxing and will decrease your inflammation! It's so anti-inflammatory thanks to how it boosts the magnesium levels in the body. Higher levels of magnesium have been linked to boosting energy and alleviating insomnia or restlessness at night.[1] It also naturally detoxes you, and can soothe muscle and joint inflammation almost instantly, as well as reduce swelling. This is especially important for recovery if you're working out a lot or you're an athlete, or if you've been feeling some achy joint pain.

MAGGIE'S GO-TO SOAK

1. First, fill your bathtub with warm water, at the temperature that you desire.
2. As the bathtub is filling, "set the scene" a little bit! Light some candles, put on some gentle music, grab a good book, or even turn on a good show.
3. Add 1 to 2 cups of Epsom salts to your bath plus 4 drops of eucalyptus essential oil, 3 drops of cinnamon essential oil, and 2 drops of lemon essential oil. These are all immune-boosting oils that will keep your health on point.
4. Slowly submerge yourself in the water! This is where I like to do a visualization technique. Close your eyes and imagine that the Epsom salts are drawing the toxins out of your body. Imagine your leukocyte soldier friends feeling stronger and ready to work as the toxins are drawn out. Take some deep, grounding breaths and orient yourself in the present moment, feeling how nice the warm water feels, and feeling gratitude for a few moments of relaxation. Trust that as you turn to total relaxation, the Epsom salts will continue to work their magical powers, helping your body to detox!
5. Soak for 20 minutes or up to one hour while enjoying your book, music, show, or continued visualization. You can even do your lymphatic massage while you're in the bath to be time-efficient, while sipping on your lemon water or a cup of matcha tea, of course!

LYMPHATIC MASSAGE

Here's how I like to think of it: the lymphatic system is essentially the "trash can" of our body. It exists to help the body get rid of everything that we don't need anymore, which also means it *holds* everything that we don't need anymore, and it can easily get backed up with all the toxins and waste. So, lymphatic massages help us drain the toxins and buildup in the lymphatic system and its tissues properly and more quickly than it can do on its own. This can help to fight off infection and reduce water retention—if you've ever gotten off a flight after a long day of traveling and noticed your face was a bit puffy, this is a sign that your lymphatic system has been blocked! Massage coming right up!

Most people think of the face when they think of lymphatic massages, but there are also whole-body lymphatic drainage massages available. These help the lymphatic system to drain what it doesn't need anymore, which leads to a decrease in inflammation and swelling throughout the body, and it can also boost the body's immune system. It's important to do some form of a lymphatic drainage massage every single day—because it's as important as taking the trash out! You would never forget to take the trash out for days.

Imagine what you want the inside of your body to look like and feel like. First, imagine a worn-down home that hasn't opened the windows or had a deep clean in forever. It's covered in mold, trash is overflowing, the carpet is stained, dirt has been trekked in, and the space smells and feels toxic and dirty! Gross.

Now imagine a home that's beautiful, chic, organized, and clean. It's spotless! It smells fresh and wonderful, and the sun comes streaming in through the clear windows. Everything is in its place, as if a deep spring clean has just been completed and you love your space once again. I always feel like I can be far more productive and have a much better day when I'm living and working in a clean space. Your body's cells feel the same!

You have a choice which "home" environment you want the inside of your body to mimic. By doing lymphatic massage, you're getting rid of all the trash, dirt, stains, mold, and bacteria in that first home, and restoring your home to its sacred and clean state! Think of this as a daily habit, and to make it easier to implement, "habit stack it" (a principle from James Clear's book *Atomic Habits*) with another regular part of your day.[2] For example: if you always wash your face right after you wake up, "stack" in the habit of doing a facial lymphatic massage right after you dry your face. You're likely going to put on moisturizer anyway, so have a spa moment with it. A lymphatic massage feels nice and has marked benefits, so it's a fun and easy habit to implement. You may even see visible changes to your face and its puffiness immediately after the massage (major bonus for a morning meeting or photo shoot)!

This lymphatic massage can be done on your face with an all-natural, nontoxic oil or lotion, and you can use a chi roller, a natural jade roller, or a gua sha stone. I use a natural jade roller and oil from a health food store (my favorite personal face oils right now are Annmarie skin care and Mad Hippie). I put a little bit of oil on my face, then get to work with the jade roller! I begin on my neck, then do my cheeks from my chin outward, and then go outward from the middle of my nose on both sides. You can use your favorite moisturizer or vitamin E oil (all-natural ingredients, please!) and rub it over your face and neck.

Jade rollers also have a smaller side, and I use that for right underneath my eyes. I also sometimes use a Clarisonic facial cleanser, which has a massage head that gently vibrates. I'll go over those same areas that I do with a jade roller with the Clarisonic massage head, which also works as a lymphatic massage.

DRY BRUSHING

Dry brushing is another great way to lightly exfoliate your skin all over your body and promote circulation, *and* it's thought to have an energizing effect! A dry brush is a wooden brush with tougher bristles that can be massaged over your body with a little bit of oil. While the bristles can be a bit rougher, it should never hurt or scratch the skin. Rather, it should be the right mix of soft and rough that helps the body detoxify and assists in more lymph drainage. The idea is to rub the brush upward, *toward* your heart space.

I recommend dry brushing one to two times a week only—it's important to give your skin a break because of the rougher bristles and the exfoliation component. Also, wash your dry brush between uses because dry skin flakes can build up in the bristles. True to its name and easy to remember, make sure to dry brush when your skin is dry—not while in the shower, in the bath, or immediately after you get out of either.

SUPERCHARGE YOUR SLEEP

Sleep must be a priority to keep your immune system strong. I always noticed in college that after I'd pull an all-nighter studying for an exam or staying up way too late on the weekends, my body would feel run-down. And run-down it was! Sleep is beyond necessary for helping your immune system work effectively. In fact, it's when you go to bed that the immune system can do its best work.

During your waking hours, when you're up and moving around and eating and working, your body is juggling a *lot*. Plus, you're more prone to stress when you're awake, even from situations like a long wait at the supermarket when you're running late for your next phone call. These periods of mental stress and exposure to outdoor stressors (such as car exhaust, a fellow shopper's strong cologne, or a mosquito bite) are disruptive to the immune system, because they tug at the immune system's attention in a hundred different directions. Think about the last time that you were trying to work on something, but everything that was happening around you distracted you: your kids needed help with their homework, the fire alarm went off, the phone rang twice, the dog wouldn't stop barking, and the thermostat needed adjusting!

Just as we need peace and quiet to get into our flow state for our best work, our leukocytes do, too. That's why our sleep is so important. It's when all the noise shuts off and they can get to work!

Particularly, when we go to sleep, our immune system is able to signal additional helpers called cytokines. These help further with fighting against disease and infection. When you get less sleep, cytokines aren't released as readily, which can take a toll on your immune system. That's why sleep should be sacred!

MAGGIE'S MELATONIN-MOVING NIGHTTIME ROUTINE

Part of getting a great night's sleep is preparing with a nighttime routine. No matter how tired you are, jumping immediately from staring into the blue light of your cell phone and eating a late-night snack into forcing yourself to fall asleep is challenging. So, here's my melatonin-moving nighttime routine:

1. At least one hour before bed, put away all electronics. Instead, opt for a good read or conclude the day with some journaling.
2. Dim all the lights in your house. This signals to the body that it's bedtime, as you'll remember from the last chapter. Continuing to use bright lights can confuse your body, making it think it's daytime! Use reddish-tinted lights, or turn the lights down.
3. Finish eating a few hours prior to bed, so that your digestive system isn't working so hard when your head hits the pillow.

4. Stick to a consistent bedtime routine. If your bedtime is 10:30 every night, hold yourself accountable to put electronic devices away at 9:30 every night.

5. Make your bedtime routine more like a "ritual." Our bodies respond well to habits. By saying, "It's time to go to sleep now," and getting into your cozy cocoon of a bed at the same time every evening, your internal body clock is more likely to get with the program.

6. Say to yourself before you go to sleep, "As I close my eyes, I know my body will fall into a wonderful night of deep, regenerative sleep. I will sleep restfully and peacefully, supporting my body and immune system in its wonderful work to keep me safe, vibrant, and healthy! I thank my body for the work it does for me daily, and look forward to waking up in the morning refreshed and strong." Write that out on a card and keep it on your bed stand to read each night. You can also make your own version of this little mantra as you see fit. Setting the intention for a healing night of restful sleep is more helpful than you know!

Finally, I'll add that your mood greatly impacts your immune system's ability to fight for you. For example, fear, worry, and anxiety will actually decrease your immune system and make it even more likely for you to get sick. Supercharging your immune system is about helping it the same way it helps us, by giving it the proper positive inputs—sleep, mood, nutrition, movement—for it to do its best work!

12

EXERCISE AND MOVEMENT

Healing requires a holistic, all-systems approach. Beyond diet, elimination of environmental stressors, and mindset, another nonnegotiable to help your body reach its optimal state is to *get moving*!

Just as when you don't use your brain frequently, you can lose memory and some intellectual functionality, the same thing happens when your body sits idle for too long. It needs blood flow and exercise to work in the way that it was intended to work. Countless studies prove the power of physical activity in preventing diseases and boosting moods. Research from the *Canadian Medical Association Journal* stated that "physical inactivity is a modifiable risk factor for cardiovascular disease and a widening variety of other chronic diseases, including diabetes mellitus, cancer (colon and breast), obesity, hypertension, bone and joint diseases (osteoporosis and osteoarthritis), and depression."[1]

That's one long list. The study went on to report that women who did intensive exercise saw a 20–30% reduction in their risk for breast cancer as opposed to their inactive counterparts, and men and women saw a 30–40% reduction in their risk for colon cancer. Weight-bearing exercise increases the mineral bone density, so those who did more resistance weight training were less at risk of developing osteoporosis. Regular exercise can also contribute to mood, and research has shown time and time again that physical activity can alleviate some of the devastating symptoms of anxiety and depression.[2]

I cannot overstate the importance of some form of movement. However, it's important to really recognize which "movement" is best for you at the current time, and not to overstress yourself if you're in a state of severe inflammation. For example, I have clients who come to me with severe internal imbalances and fatigue who wake up and start each day on "empty," and they can hardly make it around the block for an afternoon stroll. That's OK! And I urge you to please not push yourself. In these cases, I recommend that you do small movements walking around the house. Every few hours, just walk around your house or even just do a few bodyweight squats, swing your arms, or do yoga-type movements at your desk. Low-impact bodyweight Pilates is also a great option!

The more you can move, the better—even if the movements seem small and like they won't add up to much. It still gets your circulation flowing, your digestion moving, and can aid against inflammation. So, start slow. Maybe exercising first thing in the morning isn't the best way to go for you if you wake up feeling depleted. Instead, begin the day with an anti-inflammatory smoothie (recipes in the next chapter!) or a good juice, then try to get moving a little later in the day when your energy is up a bit. However you can move, do it!

When we move, it increases the communication channels between the brain and the body through the brain signals. If you've been sitting all day, the brain isn't too sure what's going on in the body. Think of movement as a way to get everything in sync. In fact, right now as you're reading, lift your arms to the sky, then bend slightly side to side to bring a nice stretch throughout your body. Even that helps! These brain signals are crucial for digestion and getting your bowels moving, which will help to detoxify and cleanse the body. Just get moving.

CHOOSE AN EXERCISE YOU LOVE

Now, I'm not at all saying that you have to join a high intensity–style gym, push yourself with interval training daily, or train for a marathon (unless of course you're feeling great and looking to further your athletic performance in a safe way). The type of movement you do really depends on your current health status, and how each different movement makes you feel—not just physically but also mentally. If you woke up early this morning to run on the treadmill and hated every second of it, it actually would be doing more harm than good. It would stress you out with every minute, elevating you into the sympathetic nervous system. Then, tomorrow, when it would be time to get out of bed and do it again, you could feel your skin crawl. That's no way to start a new habit! It is crucial that you enjoy your exercise.

A study from the *International Journal of Behavioral Nutrition and Physical Activity* evaluated the impact of intrinsic motivation on exercise.[3] Think of an exercise you really just do not enjoy—never have and likely never will. Now, contrast that with an exercise you really enjoy. Imagine those two types of exercise in your head right now . . . really think about them both. What do you dislike, and what doesn't bring you joy? Do you have the picture? Now, what lights you up inside, leaves you feeling amazing, and makes you look forward to doing it? You may feel a different level of energy in your body for each. One makes you want to go back to bed. One makes you excited! Those neurotransmitters that are released in response to your thought about doing each type of exercise are either negative or positive. Positive neurotransmitters are beyond powerful in healing your body, decreasing inflammation, and leading you to see the results that you're seeking. In other words, just by enjoying your exercise and getting excited about doing it, you're already sparking benefits.

A note here, because I know there are probably some of you reading this who felt a bit lost on that last question since you *don't* like to exercise. None of it! Or right now you're so depressed or in pain that you can't even get out of bed and it takes all your energy just to go to the bathroom and maybe (probably not) brush your hair that day. You can't even fathom moving your body in any possible way, even in a lighter way like a walk. I hear you and I'm listening. So, what is something you enjoy that involves some type of movement? If you're bedridden today maybe you don't move much, but let's focus on the other days. I had one of my clients just focus on walking once a day from her bed down her hallway while she listened to her favorite song. She just had to be up and walking during that song. If she then felt motivated and up for it, she would hit "next" to hear the next song, and so forth. All just right in her hallway. I'm OK with baby steps, I'm just not OK with no steps—I am not going to let you pick up this book and NOT finally make a change to get your life back. I'm here for you!

If there's no workout you enjoy, find a song you enjoy to tie any tiny movement to. That excitement—the song, the fitness routine—causes intrinsic motivation, which matters greatly. The study found that intrinsic motivation was far more predictive of long-term exercise adherence. Remember, we're going for the long game here, with the complete adoption of exercise habits. This isn't going to be a two-week detox and workout program that will heal you forever—that doesn't exist. It needs to be consistent. So, long-term exercise in your lifestyle is paramount. What excites you enough that you can see yourself doing it three times a week every week from here on out? What excites you enough to become the person who does that thing? People will just know you love to dance, or hike, or run, or lift, or all of the above! Become that person. Love and enjoy the process of moving your body in a way that heals and comes from a place of love and nourishment, and you'll see results beyond measure.

Luckily, we've never lived in a time with more fitness options. There are countless class options, from Pilates to spin class to water aerobics! Many of these options are accessible from your home, such as yoga instructors with hundreds of videos on YouTube, or Nike's new app for at-home workouts. A stationary bike is another great way to get a sweat in from home, and many bikes allow you to tune in with others from across the globe who are also cycling! I encourage you to have some fun trying all of them out. Remember that nothing is going to be easy from the get-go, but if you try it a few times and consistently enjoy it, consider signing up! Get together with some friends to try the classes, or if you think you're better on your own terms, create a habit of going for a jog every morning as the sun rises or an evening walk with your family. My husband, kids, and I walk around the neighborhood almost every evening and I've come to really look forward to it. The more consistently you show up for yourself and your movement and do it in a way that you enjoy, the better!

Don't be afraid to switch it up, either. Maybe on the weekend you go for a long bike ride, whereas during the week you stay at home and follow an online yoga workout. Research has shown that exercise should hit four main categories: strength, endurance, flexibility, and balance.[4] So, in your yoga exercises, you're likely hitting on flexibility, balance, and a little bit of strength. But on a long bike ride, you're capturing more of that endurance aspect (with a bit of balance, especially if you're biking over rocky terrain!).

Recent research has also found that doing exercises in synchrony with others can boost self-esteem.[5] In classes where participants go through a vinyasa flow or similar exercises at the same timing, while following an instructor, can result in simply making you feel better! Don't overcomplicate this, though. If you personally don't love working out in a big room full of other people, you can also find synchrony following an instructor's recommendations through an online program, or just by taking a long walk with your friends.

Aside from all these benefits of exercise, research has also found that cardiovascular exercise can be anti-inflammatory. *Aging and Disease* journal reported that "studies have demonstrated that regularly performed cardiovascular exercise training may reduce markers of systemic inflammation."[6]

Specifically, "regular exercise reduces fat mass and adipose tissue inflammation which is known to contribute to systemic inflammation . . . exercise also increases muscle production of IL-6 which is known to . . . increase anti-inflammatory cytokines." In addition, "Exercise training also increases vagal tone which according to the cholinergic anti-inflammatory reflex . . . could lead to reductions in systemic inflammation."

So there you have it—the tandem benefits of exercise can only help. Start slow and do what you most enjoy. This is all supposed to be fun and it can be!

QUICK TIPS FOR STARTING EXERCISE

Below are some tips on the types of exercise based on your inflammation type. This is most applicable in your initial healing stages. Once you're well, long-term—do what makes you feel best!

MUSCLE AND JOINT INFLAMMATION

Opt for low-impact movements. Heavy lifting and high-intensity interval training are not your friend. Swimming, yoga, and Pilates are fantastic options to get movement on point, decrease inflammation, increase circulation, and do no further harm to your body. Time to take a break from the intensity!

HORMONAL INFLAMMATION AND THE THYROID

Your adrenal glands are likely in the tank. Your thyroid isn't firing properly. Your hormones are off. You are on "E," my friend. You cannot be pushing yourself in the gym too hard right now. Your joints and muscles are pretty much fine, though, so your best option would be lifting weights for middle-rep movements. This might look like one exercise being 8–12 reps of a standing dumbbell curl x 3 sets. What you're not doing is high-intensity training, which would look like 8–12 dumbbell curl reps with 20 burpees between each set. High-intensity training, although useful in certain situations, is not going to help you with healing at this time.

INFLAMMATION CAUSED BY SUGAR

You're good to go with a variety of workouts. In fact, high-intensity workouts are going to be helpful in rebalancing your sugar levels. You can't not work out. Every day, 30 minutes a day, I want you to be getting in some sort of sweat. You can do this!

PSYCHOLOGICAL STRESS

If you've been struggling with anxiety and anxious feelings, research has shown that regular aerobic exercise can bring you out of the sympathetic nervous system state and therefore relieve the fight-or-flight stress response in the body.[7] Or, if you have both anxiety and depression, research has also found that meditative movement can help.[8] If you have depression right now, depending on the severity, a walk outside may be your best recommendation, or simply zoning out to a great playlist while lifting weights. If you're in a depressive state that has you cooped up at home all day under blankets, I hear you—all I want you to do is simply walk around the house. Get up and moving various times throughout the day, and hopefully the next day you'll feel up for pushing yourself to get to that walk outdoors—it will be worth it!

DIGESTIVE INFLAMMATION

If you're bloated or constipated, cardiovascular fitness will be very useful—treadmill, bike, stairs, a walk outside. If you're having diarrhea, it's the opposite. For those with active diarrhea, I'd recommend weight lifting with free weights or the machines at a gym. I don't need you running around outside feeling stabbing pains in your abdomen or like you're going to poop your pants in front of everyone at the gym. On days of diarrhea flares, simply choose basic fitness options such as sitting dumbbell bicep curls. You still need cardiovascular activity, but choose a day or time when your bowels are a little more at ease. At-home fitness is also a great option for those with digestive inflammation. You're at home, so you can easily get to the bathroom or attend to your digestive distress alone. Yoga, Pilates video, cycle, even a cardio video from home would be great.

ALLERGIES, ASTHMA, AND SKIN INFLAMMATION

If you have active allergies and asthma, your trigger will determine if you ought to exercise indoors at a gym, at home, or outdoors. It may be that in your own home, with nontoxic products, is the best option for you. Gyms use a lot of toxic chemicals to clean their equipment in an attempt to keep us healthy, but for your body, this may not be the case. The fragrances and toxins may flare your symptoms and lead to headaches and skin rashes. Outdoors may make symptoms flare up if you have allergies to things like pollen. Skin inflammation does not typically impair your ability to do any sort of fitness, so feel free to focus on what you love most!

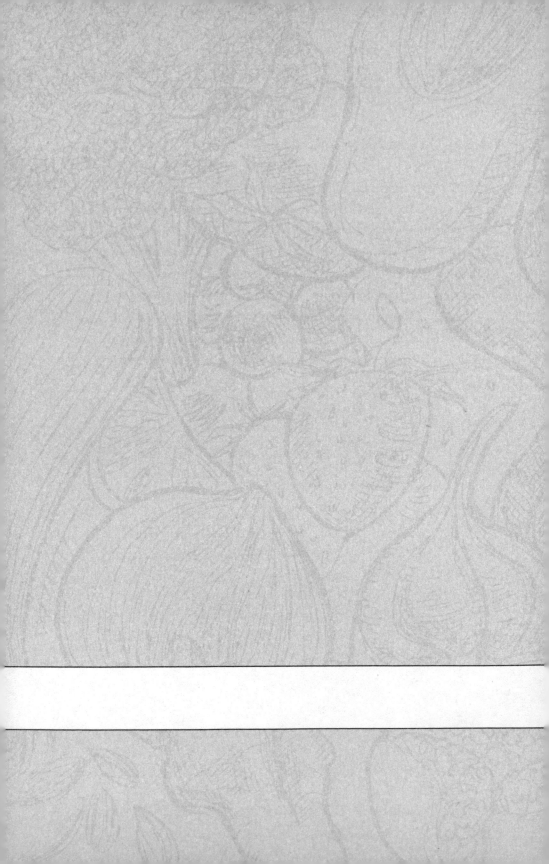

EAT TO TREAT

13

YOUR ANTI-INFLAMMATORY PANTRY AND FRIDGE

As we've discussed extensively throughout this book, much of what causes inflammation is your diet. In chapter 5 we talked about sugar and how the standard American diet includes far too much of it. We'll dive further into processed foods and the chemicals within them that can cause inflammation in your gut, and corresponding inflammation through the rest of your body. Food is fuel! We should eat to feel good and give our bodies the best chance at natural energy, natural healing, and natural vibrancy, rather than adding the sticky sugar, white flour, and processed food "gunk" to our machines.

It's worth restating that your gut is, essentially, your second brain. Because of the enteric nervous system, what goes through your digestive system has a direct impact on your mood, your endocrine system and the hormones that are released, your skin, and your joints. It's all interconnected—and it starts with what you're putting inside your body!

Make the decision that right here, right now, you're going to change your whole life. THIS is the moment you'll look back on and talk about in five, ten, fifteen years down the road. The moment you took your life into your own hands and transformed into your very best self. You built resilience. You tried new things. You fully loved yourself. You evolved. You can do this!

GROCERY STORE MANTRA

Eating anti-inflammatory foods begins with how you choose to grocery shop—where you make the purchases to fill your home with! Rather than making a strict "grocery list," I have always loved the idea of having a "grocery store mantra." This is what you repeat to yourself as you wander through the store and make choices for the week ahead. Remember, mindset comes first for making lifelong changes!

Grocery shopping should be fun! It's an opportunity to find real, whole foods that will naturally energize you and fill you up. Your mantra will ensure that every trip to the grocery store is an act of self-love, where you feel like you're giving more to your best self each time you choose an item to put in your cart.

Here are some grocery store mantras you can use. Choose one that resonates (or shake it up and use a different one for each grocery store trip), and feel free to customize it for your specific goals:

- I eat real, whole food.
- I eat to nourish my body.
- I eat to feel vibrant and naturally energized.
- The food choices I make are acts of self-love.
- I eat to feed my health and vibrancy.
- My food choices determine how I feel.
- Real food nourishes my body.

These can be customized to your goals by adding in what real, nourishing food will help you to do. For example:

- I fuel my body with real food so I'm always at the top of my game in my business.
- I eat real, nutritious foods to fuel my body to meet my athletic goals.
- I love giving my body the nutrition it needs to be in its full vibrancy—which gives me a radiant glow and beautiful skin!
- I eat well to show my children a great example of honoring your body through real food.
- I show my body how much I love and appreciate it through the real food that I give it, and it returns the love to me as it heals its [insert symptom here].

When you use a mantra to get your mind in the right place for grocery shopping, your cart will fill up with more nutritious items, and maybe, just maybe, you'll have a big smile on your face while enjoying a peaceful trip to the store. Contrast this with having anxiety and stress filling your mind, which could easily lead to autopilot taking over as you fill your cart with the same old unhealthy items.

BASICS OF YOUR GROCERY TRIP

When at the grocery store, focus on the outer perimeter of the store. This is where the fruits, vegetables, and more natural products are found. Toward the center of the store will tend to be the aisles with the packaged and processed foods, including items with added preservatives and chemicals in them that allow them to be "shelf stable" for long periods of time. The more you can stick to the outer perimeter, the less you'll be tempted to pick up a packaged snack while you're walking by, or even opt for an "organic" or "healthy" option that really isn't as healthy as it's being marketed to be.

Even if you're in your neighborhood's natural food store and it's a package of organic cheddar chips, I urge you to still avoid it! Another general rule of thumb is to buy items from the refrigerated section. They most likely are healthier for you than the items on the unrefrigerated shelves that you THEN put in the fridge when you get home. For example: hummus, mayo, and guacamole will be best and freshest if you find them in the refrigerated section of the store as opposed to the shelf. If you find that item in a jar in one of the middle aisles, it's more likely it could have added chemicals and ingredients you don't typically want to eat.

In general, choose to fill your cart with mostly vegetables. And be sure that those veggies are a variety of colors to boost the phytonutrients your body is getting from them. Each different color indicates a different nutrient makeup, and they're all highly beneficial for various reasons. For example: if you always purchase orange carrots, this time try purple carrots! Or swap your go-to green bell pepper for the red. A varied and diverse diet full of plants is one that will decrease inflammation and lead to endless health benefits. When choosing your items, I do recommend opting for "organic" to lessen the amount of chemicals your body is exposed to. It's a simple swap that can go a long way.

PANTRY RESET

One fun project to kick-start your anti-inflammatory lifestyle is to do a total pantry reset. Set aside a few hours to go through every item you have in your pantry, knowing that it's actually going to end up pretty empty! When you first look, you likely have leftover snack boxes, processed foods, canned items, spices from years ago, and more. An anti-inflammatory lifestyle focuses on foods that are usually kept in the fridge, so you'll only have a few staple pantry items once the reset is over. It will feel SO good to have that pantry wiped clean and refreshed—I'm sure of it!!

In regard to what *not* to get at the store specifically, there are what I call the "Triple Trouble" I personally abide by and ask my clients to remove from their diet as they begin working with me. These three trouble foods have been found to cause the most complications in my clients with symptoms and auto-immune disease. When we remove these three foods, we knock down inflammation in a tremendous way from the very start and help our body to heal itself quickly. It makes your life so much easier to just get these out of the math equation we're trying to solve! Yes, it may feel scary to remove these things at first, but it is so worth it when you can feel better than you have in years—decades!—from a short-term removal of the below while we rebalance the body. The Triple Trouble items are:

- Dairy
- Sugar
- Grains (even gluten-free!)

I know this can seem restrictive and prescriptive. It's almost counterintuitive to what I preach, since I always say there is no "one-size-fits-all" diet approach. However, from consistent clinical experience and research, I know that if you really want to up-level your health and see major changes, taking out or greatly reducing these three foods will accelerate your efforts. An important mental adjustment is to move away from the "Ugh, I'm only going to be eating *healthy* from now on," or "But I'll miss out on X, Y, and Z," or "But I want to enjoy my life." *This mentality is from a place of fear and scarcity, and it needs to shift.* Rather, this should and can be an empowering switch. This is going to be fun, amazing, exciting! You are going to feel so great and you'll finally feel fully alive. Everyone will notice the amazing changes you're making, and you may inspire them to join in as they witness the progress you're making in your life and its impact on your life.

You don't have to eliminate every single canned and packaged item in your pantry, but you do want those few staples to be anti-inflammatory. In alignment with a truly anti-inflammatory pantry, most of you will be ditching your previous go-to pantry items in this removal process!

Begin by removing most of your items that are canned (they're canned in aluminum, which is not healthy anyway, even if the label reads "BPA free"), highly processed, packaged with added chemicals and toxic ingredients, or that have sugar, dairy, or grains as an ingredient. And don't just remove them from the pantry or put them in their own little corner or bin—throw them away! Simply moving your favorite snack cookies to a different place in your kitchen "just in case" you might want one is not the best idea. You must remove all distractions and temptations from your immediate environment. Get it out and start totally fresh! Keeping a food that carries all the ingredients and preservatives we're choosing to avoid in our commitment to an anti-inflammatory lifestyle and telling yourself you just won't eat it is no different than an alcoholic keeping their favorite liquor in their liquor cabinet. Lessen the temptations in your home to make it easier for you to make the healthy choice. And it will clear out the "old" to make room for the "new." In this case, the "new" is an organized, clean, fresh, and anti-inflammatory pantry that nourishes your body inside and out and symbolizes your new start! Think of every Instagram-worthy, beautiful, sparkling, clean kitchen and obsessively organized pantry. That's the goal!

Ideally, your pantry will be rid of all cereals (unless you have one of my approved anti-inflammatory options—there are few out there!), fruit snacks, soda, flour, sugar, chips, pastries, and processed bars.

ANTI-INFLAMMATORY GROCERY LIST STAPLES

These are staples for the long term. You may want to avoid certain things on this list during the immediate rebalancing phase and of course during our detox meal plan:

- **Plenty of lean proteins**, such as chicken, salmon, and turkey.
- **Colorful arrays of vegetables!** The more color you can get on a plate, the better. Fill your pantry with bell peppers, onions, asparagus, broccoli, cauliflower, carrots, okra— any vegetables that stand out to you.
- **Fresh fruit.** Think: citrus fruits like limes and lemons (especially lemons for lemon detox water!), antioxidant-rich berries like blueberries, and apples.
- If you're doing grains, choose **gluten-free grains**, like rice, oats, and quinoa.
- **Seasonings and flavors that are certifiably anti-inflammatory**, such as cinnamon, cacao powder, and turmeric.
- **Nut milks** like almond milk or cashew milk. Just be sure to read the label to confirm that they don't have added artificial or synthetic ingredients.
- **Nut butters.** Again, read the label!
- **Healthy fats** such as avocados, extra-virgin olive oil, nuts, seeds, and coconut oil.

FOOD INGREDIENTS TO AVOID

I value simplicity and real, whole foods—as you can see from the list of pantry staples! So, anything that doesn't seem to echo that same simplicity might be best left on the store shelf. Nowadays, even a simple box of crackers can have so many suspicious ingredients that can cause inflammation flare-ups. An easy rule of thumb is simply to not purchase anything that has ingredients that sound like long chemical names when you check the back of the box or bag. If you think one or a multiple of the ingredients could belong in a chemistry textbook, leave it behind! Many of my clients and friends feel better knowing exactly what to look out for, just because so many of today's packaged and processed foods have preservatives and chemicals that we don't even know can be harmful. So, for your use, the following is a full list of ingredients to avoid in processed and packaged foods.[1] If you run up against a nutritional list on a package that you just don't know for sure about, this list will answer your questions! Here's your full list of "nevers" when it comes to food ingredients:

Acesulfame potassium (Ace K) is an artificial sweetener that has been linked to cancer. It's commonly found in diet sodas, protein shakes, yogurt, and "sugar-free" products.

Artificial flavors are what make your food and drink taste like something else—like what makes a sports drink have a "cherry" flavor. Any artificial flavor can have up to one hundred ingredients and are ridden with chemicals and preservatives.

Artificial sweeteners have been reported to contribute to weight gain by stimulating your appetite and increasing sugar cravings. Look out for anything labeled "low-calorie," "sugar-free," "reduced-sugar," or "diet."

Aspartame is commonly found in artificial sweeteners and has been linked to the increased risk of heart disease, leukemia, brain tumors, and lymphomas. It can be found in fruit cups, protein shakes, diet sodas, and anything that says "sugar-free."

Azodicarbonamide (also sometimes referred to as "yoga mat chemical") is a dough conditioner (in many sandwich breads and other baked goods) that the World Health Organization has linked to allergies and asthma.

BHA (butylated hydroxyanisole) is a synthetic preservative that disrupts the endocrine system and has been linked to cancer. It's what preserves foods like canned soup, potato chips, sausage, pepperoni, spaghetti sauce, and more.

BHT (butylated hydroxytoluene) is a synthetic preservative that can affect the way the gut signals to the brain that the body is full. It's also been linked to cancer and can disrupt the endocrine system. It preserves foods like packaged nuts and cake mixes.

Blue 1 (Brilliant Blue) is an artificial blue dye made from petroleum. The FDA specifically found that it can turn colons bright blue, can cause refractory hypotension and metabolic acidosis, and can increase the risk of kidney tumors. This blue dye is commonly found in fruit snacks, candy, popsicles, and gum.

Calcium peroxide is a bleach and dough conditioner that is heavily processed and has been banned in Europe, China, and some natural food stores in the United States. It can cause eye, skin, and respiratory irritation.

Calcium propionate is a mold inhibitor that, according to the *Journal of Pediatric Child Health*, may lead to restlessness and sleep disturbance in children. It's found in croutons, bread, and baked goods, and can also damage the stomach lining in adults.

Canola oil is a refined cooking oil in frozen meals, dressings, snacks, and sauces. Its refining process includes contamination from many chemical solvents, bleaches, neutralizers, and deodorizers. The biggest risk is its inclusion of the neurotoxin hexane from the refining process.

Caramel color is brown food coloring found in pancake syrup, drinks at coffee shops, deli meats, sodas, and cereals. It's created by heating ammonia and sulfites, and in 2014 the Consumers Union petitioned the FDA to require manufacturers to list caramel color as an ingredient and ban it from any natural foods.

Carrageenan is a thickening agent found in coconut milk, cottage cheese, coffee creamers, dairy-free milk, ice cream, almond milk, soy milk, and deli meats. It can lead to digestive inflammation and consequent digestive problems.

Cellulose is another thickener used in some shredded cheeses, spice mixes, pancake syrup, and foods that say "high fiber" or "added fiber." It can lead to inflammation, digestive issues, and weight gain.

Citric acid is a preservative and a flavor that gives a sour taste. It's added to some energy drinks, citrus sodas, bottled iced teas, canned tomatoes, candy, flavored chips, and baby food. Citric acid is actually natural when it comes from lemons, but the additive for its use in packaged foods can lead to tooth decay and an irritated digestive system.

Corn oil is a refined cooking oil that presents the same danger as canola oil from its refining process and the neurotoxin hexane. It can be found in microwave popcorn, snack mixes, coated pretzels, sausages, and chips and cookies.

Corn syrup is sugar made from corn that's been heavily processed. The GMO corn used for its production usually produces its own insecticide.

Cottonseed oil is another refined cooking oil that comes from cotton crops. Because of the great number of pesticides sprayed on cotton, cottonseed oil typically has trace amounts of pesticides and goes through more chemical refining with hexane and bleach.

DATEM (diacetyl tartaric acid esters of monoglycerides) is a dough conditioner that comes from canola oil or soybean oil, and is usually found in baked goods, crackers, and bread. It can be a source of highly dangerous trans fat, which is the type of fat that can be quite harmful if eaten regularly. Trans fats can increase your "bad" cholesterol and lead to heart complications. There really are no benefits of trans fats, so it's best to reduce.

Dextrose is another heavily processed form of sugar from corn, similar to corn syrup. It presents the same danger because of the GMO corn. It's commonly found in meat sticks, frozen meals, chips, and cake mixes.

Dimethylpolysiloxane is an ingredient used in Silly Putty and . . . French fries? It's also found in yogurt, deep-fried foods, and fountain drinks. It's a defoaming agent that isn't allowed to be used in milk.

Enriched and **bleached flour** are heavily processed flours in sandwich bread and baked goods. Since these flours have no nutritional value on their own, synthetic vitamins are added. The wheat used to make them is usually sprayed with toxic herbicide.

Erythritol is a sugar alcohol and sweetener that can have a detrimental effect on the digestive system. Sugar alcohols are a sugar substitute that promote fewer calories and carbs than regular sugar. However, sugar alcohols such as erythritol may disturb the microbiota of the gut, and can lead to diarrhea and headaches even from normal amounts. It's found in diet drinks, pudding cups, yogurt, and Stevia products.

High fructose corn syrup (HFCS) and **fructose corn syrup**. Fructose (HFCS-90) and fructose syrup contain even more fructose than high fructose corn syrup. Too much of either can lead to cardiovascular disease, high blood sugar, and obesity. They can be found in soft drinks, ketchup, cookies, cereal, yogurt, granola bars, and frosting.

Maltodextrin is a heavily processed starch that works as a sweetener, preservative, and thickener. It disturbs the gut's microbiota, and is found in frozen meals, pudding, mac and cheese, and powdered drink mixes.

Monoglycerides and **diglycerides** are emulsifiers that keep ingredients together, found commonly in ice cream sandwiches, peanut butter, nondairy creamers, bread, and tortillas. These both contain artificial trans fats and can contribute to an increased risk of type 2 diabetes and heart disease. The CDC has linked them to at least twenty thousand heart attacks each year.

Monosodium glutamate is an artificial flavor enhancer in dressings, soups, frozen meals, and chips. It's created to promote food cravings to make you eat more, and can lead to depression, headaches, and obesity.

Natural flavors are made from chemicals derived from anything in nature—which is their only difference from artificial flavor. They too can have up to one hundred ingredients, including excitotoxins to get you to keep eating. They're in almost all processed foods.

Neotame is a new artificial sweetener that may be more harmful than aspartame. It can be found in gum, diet juices or sodas, drink mixes, and orange drink.

Partially hydrogenated oils have been solidified with chemical processing and are usually made with other harmful oils such as GMO soybean, cottonseed, or canola oil. They can lead to an increased risk of diabetes and heart disease, and are commonly found in cookies, crackers, baked goods, and nondairy creamers.

Propyl gallate is another synthetic preservative that can increase the risk of tumors and endocrine disruption. It can be found in sausage, stuffing mix, and pizza.

Propylparaben and **methylparaben** are synthetic preservatives that are endocrine disruptors, leading to reproductive issues and breast cancer. They are found in tortillas, frosting, and snack cakes.

Red #3 (erythrosine) is an artificial dye derived from petroleum. Even though it's been banned from cosmetics, it's currently still permitted in food. It's in maraschino cherries, sausage casings, candy, and strawberry milk.

Red 40 (Allura Red) is another red dye from petroleum, and is the most popular artificial color in the US. In Europe, food that has Red 40 must have a warning label that says, "May Have an Adverse Effect on Activity and Attention in Children." It's in popsicles, cereal bars, soft drinks, cherry filling, fruit cups, ice cream, and more.

Sodium benzoate and **potassium benzoate (E211 and E212)** are synthetic preservatives that can produce benzene—a known carcinogen—when combined with ascorbic acid or erythorbic acid. They are found in syrups, pickles, sauces, soft drinks, and salad dressings.

Sodium nitrate and **sodium nitrite (E251 and E250)** are synthetic preservatives in deli meats, hot dogs, sausage, bacon, and meat snacks, and can increase the risk of cancer.

Sodium phosphate is a preservative you might eat daily. It's in cooked chicken, frozen desserts, frozen meals, imitation cheese slices, pudding, canned soup, and more. Frequent consumption can lead to an increased risk for chronic kidney disease, heart disease, and accelerated aging.

Soybean oil (vegetable oil) has been linked to the risk of obesity, cardiovascular disease, autoimmune diseases, inflammation, and cancer. It usually has residue from the herbicide glyphosate, which the WHO named a probable carcinogen. It's found in salad dressings, crackers, trail mix, soup, sauces, cookies, and frozen meals.

Soy protein isolate is a protein supplement made from soy flour that can lead to hormonal interruptions. It may also have residue from the carcinogen herbicide glyphosate, and is therefore linked to kidney disease, autism, and birth defects. It's found in protein powder, frozen meals, veggie burgers and veggie dogs, and protein bars.

Stevia extract (rebaudioside A or reb A) is a low-calorie sweetener that is highly processed from stevia leaves. The extraction process exposes the extract to chemicals like methanol, ethanol, and isopropanol—some of which are known carcinogens. Stevia extract is commonly found in kombucha, bottled tea, coconut water, and protein bars.

Sucralose (Splenda) is an artificial sugar that's been linked to leukemia and can also lead to weight gain. It's found in diet sodas, pudding, fruit cups, chewing gum, iced tea, and yogurt.

Synthetic vitamins are lab-created vitamins such as vitamin A palmitate, thiamine, folic acid, ascorbic acid (vitamin C), and riboflavin (vitamin B2). They are found in foods labeled as "enriched" or "fortified," and some have dangerously high levels of synthetic vitamins.

Tapioca starch replaces wheat in gluten-free foods and may spike blood sugar even more than refined sugar does.

TBHQ (tert-butylhydroquinone) is a synthetic preservative that can lead to stomach cancer, vision disturbances, child behavioral problems, and a rise in food allergies. It affects T cells in a way that can lead to allergies to shellfish, eggs, wheat, and milk. It's banned in Japan and a few other countries, and commonly found in microwave popcorn, peanut butter chocolates, biscuits, frozen pizza, and crackers.

Titanium dioxide is a food color that brightens and whitens, and can be very toxic to the body, causing cell damage. It's found in powdered sugar, marshmallows, cottage cheese, yogurt, candy, and mayonnaise.

Vanillin is an artificial flavor that imitates vanilla flavor. It can release harmful cancer-causing substances when burned.

Yellow #5 (Tartrazine – E102) and **Yellow #6 (Sunset Yellow – E110)** are artificial yellow dyes. In Europe, food that has these yellow dyes must have a warning label that says, "May Have an Adverse Effect on Activity and Attention in Children." They're found in mac and cheese, pickles, chips, candy, and fruit snacks.

See why it's best to simply eat real food and ingredients you can easily pronounce and identify?! You won't even have to worry about this list much and can know with ease that the "organic apple" you're eating is, indeed, just an organic apple.

For more on ingredients, go to maggieberghoff.com.

HELPFUL SWAPS

White, processed, or enriched flour SWAP ► **gluten-free flour, coconut flour, or almond flour**

The easiest switch to make is straight to gluten-free flour, because you can still bake according to the measurements of your favorite recipes, but simply swap out a cup of white flour for a cup of gluten-free flour. I do this all the time! I make my grandma's old recipes with this swap and no one even notices. It truly tastes no different, yet it will have a lesser inflammatory burden on your body. Coconut flour and almond flour are also wonderful choices but require different measurements, so if you're not quite ready to change up your old recipes or follow a recipe that uses these flours, stick to gluten free flour. That being said, many grain-free, sugar-free, and dairy-free recipes call for coconut flour and almond flour, so it's good to have them on hand, and I can tell you firsthand, there are the most delicious recipes out there for you to try, eliminating grains completely! Have fun experimenting with some new ways to cook and bake—an anti-inflammatory way!

Cane sugar SWAP▶ **100 percent stevia leaf or raw honey**

It doesn't matter how much you bake—the granulated, white sugar has got to go! Throw it in the trash can with all the other processed and expired pantry foods. Instead, opt for natural stevia leaf or raw honey. Both these sweeteners should be used in moderation, but they're good to have on hand when you're looking for that extra sweet taste every now and then. Again, moderation is key. Not keeping sugar in your pantry doesn't mean you'll never eat sugar again (unless you choose not to). It just means that you're choosing not to have it in your household, and not to cook and bake with it. Then, when you do have it on rare occasions, it won't be as harmful since it's not a regular or weekly thing. You'll notice an improvement in the entire family's mood, sleep, and number of sick days simply by getting rid of the sugar—try it out and report back to me with how it goes!

Semolina pasta SWAP▶ **gluten-free, red lentil pasta**

Typical pasta contains grains that can be hard to digest, is heavy in fast carbohydrates—a type of carbohydrate that releases blood glucose levels quickly and will spike your sugar levels, and can even be sprayed with toxic chemicals—all of which will lead to increased inflammation. I love using gluten-free, red lentil pasta as a replacement. It tastes great, and the red lentils have plenty of nutritional value! They're high in fiber and protein. I always have a box of it in my pantry.

Sodas SWAP▶ healthier sodas and carbonated water selections

Soda is an absolute no-no for your new lifestyle—even zero-sugar ones. Usually when you're craving a soda, it's really because you're just craving that refreshing carbonation, or it's from the habit and ritual you've built around drinking a soda. Instead, find sparkling water, or a sugar-free natural soda that uses stevia leaf for sweetener with other natural flavors. One such brand that's widely available is Zevia. This will satisfy your craving without bogging your body down with unnecessary sugar and chemicals. Ideally, I actually want you to switch to water only! No carbonation and no "healthier" sodas. However, making even this switch is a great step in the right direction—one I would be incredibly proud of you for making.

Another fun part of the pantry reset is to switch up the order of what goes where. That way, every time you look in your pantry as you kick-start your anti-inflammatory lifestyle, you'll remember your new commitment. Wipe down your shelves, and maybe even get big glass jars or new containers to hold your gluten-free flours and other items! It will look clean and new, inspiring you in your new, vibrant, and nutritious lifestyle. Can you picture it now?! Make room, Pinterest, because we have a new pantry inspiration in town.

I also make smaller switches where they're needed. For example, almost every household that frequently bakes or has kids uses food dyes. There are natural, nontoxic food dyes out there—and not just at the health food store! We recently found a great color-dye swap at Kroger that has NONE of the chemicals, sugars, or toxic ingredients. For everything you think you "need" for baking purposes or other ingredients, look for a natural version that doesn't have all the sugar and chemicals. We bake cakes, brownies, and cookies all the time, but we don't do it with chemicals. On that note, stock up on healthier dessert mixes while you're at it if that's something you're used to having! It will make your typical brownie dessert go-to so much healthier to be using a gluten-free, organic option. Simple Mills is a brand that even has grain-free and dairy-free easy dessert mixes to keep in the pantry. They have frosting, too! There's no need to use anything that's filled with chemicals that can make you sick and lead to cancer when there are nontoxic, sugar-free options available. No one will even know the difference! Imagine if every time you opened your clean and organized pantry . . . every time you opened up a cookbook to make something . . . every time you whipped up a birthday cake, you knew that everything going into your body would help heal it, decrease inflammation, and still taste absolutely amazing. Do you have a smile on your face right now imagining this? I know I sure do for you! I'm so excited for you to make these switches and experience a fuller and more vibrant, energetic life.

PANTRY STAPLES

Everyone always wants a peek behind the scenes, so I'm going to share what my personal pantry looks like here! Pantry staples I always have are:

- Rolled, gluten-free oats
- Herbs and spices such as cinnamon and turmeric (turmeric is a GREAT anti-inflammatory spice!): I add these mostly to my matcha or turmeric lattes. I also love to put these on roasted veggies.
- Chia seeds: great for throwing into smoothies.

- Flax seeds: I add them to smoothies, overnight oats, healthy pancakes or waffles, and sprinkle them on salads or cooked veggies.
- Organic protein powder made from plants or collagen: I usually have both vanilla and chocolate flavors for when I make smoothies—one of my favorite go-tos every day!
- Collagen: it is so great for your skin and gut health. It's also very anti-inflammatory and mixes easily in either hot or cold drinks. Keep individual collagen packets in the pantry as well for a quick grab when you're traveling or heading out of the house for the day, so you can add it to any drinks or even meals during the day. Add protein powder or collagen to smoothies, oats, pancake or waffle mixes, muffins, homemade bars or healthy brownies, and so much more.
- Dark chocolate: I also like to keep a few bars of dark chocolate for whenever I'm craving a sweet, after-dinner treat. It must be sugar-free, and usually is made of 85 percent dark chocolate. This sweet treat is GOOD for you because it has plenty of magnesium!
- A variety of oils: coconut oil, avocado oil, extra-virgin olive oil, and walnut oil are a few of my favorites. Use for cooking and baking. Varied and diverse—switch up the oils you always use in order to strengthen your immune system and cellular makeup, and to decrease inflammation.

SNACKS

It's worth talking about snacks, too—since that pantry reset knocked out all the typical snacks you would think of (the pretzels, chips, cookies, fruit snacks, trail mix, bars, etc.). As you make your commitment to yourself for your anti-inflammatory lifestyle, also make a commitment to snack on REAL food!

These are usually found in the fridge. This may take revamping your mindset as to what constitutes a "snack." A snack can simply be your typical meal, just a smaller potion. Make yourself a plate of veggies, a few eggs, a spoonful of raw nut butter with veggie sticks, leftover dinner, an avocado-filled almond flour wrap with meat inside, or a smoothie. Try for something with proteins, fat, and fiber to fill you up and keep your blood sugars and hormones regulated. This will boost your energy and leave you feeling amazing, as opposed to the typical "snacks" that will lead to an energy crash, brain fog, and more cravings.

The American snack diet we've eaten all our life is not conducive to refueling our body for the afternoon. And perhaps we don't even "need" that snack anyway. We've been told that it's normal to have three meals a day with snacks in between, but the reality is that this isn't necessary at all. In fact, sometimes it's actually more beneficial to eat fewer times throughout the day, so the body has longer periods to rest without needing to digest. This essentially works as a "reset."

I'll share my favorite recipes in chapter 15 (page 245) for snacks, sweet treats, breakfast, lunch, and dinner!

QUICK TIPS FOR EATING OUT

Mindset is everything. Just because you go to a restaurant does not mean you have to throw in the towel and go overboard with every single food item that will leave you feeling sick and exhausted. At the same time, going out to eat is not a time to be overly restrictive or fearful of the food. Rather, it's a fine balance between choosing what will make you feel your absolute best and honoring your choice in the moment. Then, it's about fully appreciating each bite and noticing the food, rather than hurrying through your meal and taking an "I'll start again

Monday" type of mentality. Eating anti-inflammatory is not a "diet"—it's a choice, each and every day, long-term. It's a way of life, and a value you have for yourself. It's a priority to you because you're obsessed with feeling amazing now and want to feel your best every day. Going out to eat doesn't change that a bit, unless you decide it will.

I don't believe you should stop going out to eat because you've changed your diet. There are just some easy modifications you can ask for while you're out at a restaurant with friends or family.

WHAT TO DRINK

First, let's talk about drink choices. I recommend just sticking to water. You can even bring packets of electrolytes, collagen, or greens to add to your water. If you're having coffee, skip the cream and sugar. Instead, bring along a packet of collagen to add to your cup of black coffee as a cream substitute, if you want it. Bring your own stevia rather than using the chemical-filled sweetener available at the restaurant. Just squeeze or drop it in! No one will really notice—and if they do, who cares? Confidence, remember? If you want an alcoholic beverage, check out the "cocktail" section on page 226 for my recommendations.

WHAT TO EAT

Whenever possible, choose a health-conscious restaurant. These restaurants usually label food items on the menu as "gluten-free" or "vegan." If they have this specification on the menu for a dip like hummus or guacamole, go ahead and order that if you want to—but instead of gluten-free pita bread, ask for a plate of veggies to reduce the carbohydrate overload and the likelihood of inflammatory oils. Almost every restaurant will be able to bring out a healthy plate of chopped carrots, celery, and·

cucumber sticks. You'll still love the experience of dipping into the freshly made, dairy-free dip, and you will be boosting your body with vegetables instead of bogging your body down with inflammation. If you're at a higher-end restaurant, shrimp cocktail is another great choice. You'll still feel like you're participating in the appetizer portion of the meal, but you'll do so while nourishing yourself. And while everyone else is feeling exhausted and bogged down after the meal from greasy and fried food, you'll be feeling better than ever.

You can certainly get a salad, but dress it down. "Dress it down" is really the mantra when it comes to restaurants. Usually, salads come doused in heavy dressing, cheeses, croutons, and other toppings. Ask for your salad to be gluten- and dairy-free (which will take care of most of the added toppings you don't want for anti-inflammatory living, such as croutons and cheese), and add protein if you want—grilled chicken, hard-boiled eggs, or grilled salmon. For dressing, you can just use balsamic vinegar and olive oil, or ask for a side of avocado to mash into the salad to give it a bit more flavor and add healthy fats. I'd also cut out any of the dried fruits they add, such as dried cranberries. They're just full of sugar and artificial flavorings that will lead to inflammation. If you want some fruity taste, ask for a side of real fruit to put on your salad.

For entrees, again, "dress it down." Get meat or seafood and be clear when you ask for no oil and no butter. "I'll have a chicken breast cooked without butter or oil." Easy! I used to order chicken breast with vegetables thinking I was making an anti-inflammatory choice, only to find out that it was sitting in a pool of butter for an hour before I consumed it. They can easily grill chicken without any dairy involved. Tell them that you're dairy-free. Again, stand up for what you want! You're paying for your food at this restaurant, so it should be prepared how you want to eat it (and that applies if you're not the one paying, too! If you're a restaurant customer and trusting them to cook for you, it should abide by your expectations and needs). You're likely out to eat for social reasons, but you also go out to eat to fill your body with nourishing, real foods. Bring your grocery mantra here, too, and be excited about the choices you're making right now, to lead to a healthier and happier you down the road.

Avoid items that are fried or crusted. Anything crusted is a surefire sign that it's not anti-inflammatory, because it was likely crusted with grains and butter or inflammatory vegetable oils. Sautéed is another one to stay away from. Get a side of vegetables, but make sure to ask for them steamed. Sautéed means that the vegetables were cooked in plenty of butter, cream, and oil. You want to nourish your body with the vegetables without the excess inflammation.

It's also a good idea to look at a menu ahead of time, before you actually go to the restaurant. That way, you can survey your options and plan ahead for what you're going to ask for, without feeling pressure to rush through your choice and order quickly when you're sitting at the table.

COCKTAILS

Of course, another part of going out socially or even having friends over is having cocktails or other alcoholic drinks! I personally love enjoying a drink when I'm out boating on the lake with family and friends, at a nice outdoor patio bar in the summer with my husband, or for a celebratory "cheers." You won't get the "no drinking alcohol!" rule from me. Cocktails are completely fine (in moderation, of course). They become a problem in regard to living an anti-inflammatory lifestyle when they are loaded with added sugars, artificial ingredients, glutens and grains, and chemicals. One way to decrease the odds of those added ingredients and sugars is to opt for tequila, unflavored vodka, or gin with soda water and a lime or lemon. Squeeze the lime or lemon over the drink to give it extra flavor, and you can also add in a drop or two of the stevia you brought from home to make it sweeter. Skip the syrups, sodas, and colorings. That's a clean drink!

I actually advise this clean cocktail over drinking beer or wine. Beer is inherently inflammatory and made with grains, so it bogs you down. And most wine is filled with sugars and sulfites, so I'd ditch the wine, too! If you're at home, you can easily find a sugar-free, natural wine that won't act as an inflammatory stressor when you enjoy it. There are great options on the market if you're craving that glass. I love finding a new organic, biodynamic, sugar-free wine to enjoy every now and then. Otherwise, an easy tequila, vodka, or gin with soda water is your best bet!

STICKING TO A PLAN IN REAL LIFE
A NOTE ABOUT CHANGING FOR THE BETTER

While the occasional night out can be a fun escape, to see real improvement you have to stick to a plan. If you think that switching to an anti-inflammatory lifestyle will take away your fun, freedom, and enjoyment in life, let's commit to a mindset shift. You in? In fact, living a healthy lifestyle will increase your fun, freedom, and enjoyment in life—I assure you. You'll feel energetic, vibrant, happy, stress-free, and clearheaded. You'll sleep better, be without pain, lose that stubborn weight, balance your hormones. You'll feel amazing, inside and out, and attract abundance into your life in ways you never thought possible.

I once had a client named Roger who joked he was going to be my "worst client." His daughter had found me and was hoping I could help with his health, as he was overweight and had prostate cancer. He believed somewhat in what I did, but he wasn't totally sold—mostly because he didn't want to change his lifestyle! He was retired and lived on a golf course, and he and his golfing buddies would go out to eat almost every night and drink plenty of cocktails. I didn't blame him for not wanting to completely alter his lifestyle, since it was heavily influenced by his social group and the culture of the golf course. I told him that he could absolutely make progress while still fully enjoying his lifestyle. He decided to give it a go.

We took our work slowly so he would feel comfortable, and we implemented just a few changes. We got him down to eating out only about half the amount he was used to every week. He cooked at home on the other days. We reduced his alcohol consumption (we didn't completely nix it!), and we optimized his home and cleaned up his living environment. I encouraged him to fully believe that he was going to heal his body, even without making huge drastic changes, and that this process would be fun and enjoyable. These were small changes that didn't completely topple his lifestyle and what he loved to do with his friends. But these small changes made a BIG difference.

Before we worked together, Roger had been getting monthly injections in attempts to reduce the size of the tumor in his prostate. It was staying at a consistent size. When he went in for a checkup after making those few, small changes that we had implemented together over just four months, the doctor gave him great news! His tumor had shrunk so much that he didn't even need injections anymore, and the doctor scheduled a follow-up appointment for a year later—because she didn't need to see him before that! What?! Just amazing. I've said it before and I'll say it again: the body truly does want to heal, and it will—if given a little helping hand in the right direction.

Any way that you can reduce the inflammatory stressors from your life makes a difference. When you first start to implement these changes and these swaps, you may experience some symptoms I want to make you aware of. Some of you may feel fatigued or nauseated, or experience headaches—these could be caffeine withdrawals or sugar withdrawals (which includes carbs). If you have been consuming lots of caffeine, sugar, or carbs and then you suddenly stop, it takes the body a bit of time to rebalance. That being said, you can absolutely make this shift without having these symptoms by implementing the strategies listed here.

It's important to prioritize hydration during these changes (and always!), especially because you may be dehydrated, as up to 75 percent of Americans are chronically dehydrated![2] Think of this as a detoxing process—because that's exactly what it is. Your body is finally detoxing from all the junk and chemicals that are burdening your system, and those chemicals and toxicities need a place to go. They must be removed. To expedite this and keep up with the detox process, drink water with added clean electrolyte powder, try things like visiting a sauna to sweat out more toxins, practice dry brushing, move your body, and you should ideally be having bowel movements two times a day. If you are feeling constipated or aren't hitting the twice a day mark, it's a good idea to take some type of natural prokinetic to keep things moving through your system.

Also, give your body some grace! Take an Epsom salt bath, relax more frequently, and go easy on yourself. The week you change your eating patterns shouldn't be the same week you take up a high-intensity twice-a-day workout, for example. Listen to your body, move in a way that feels good to you, take a nap when you're tired, and make sure you're getting plenty of sleep at night.

Your diet is one of the most important changes you can make to aid against inflammation, and I promise you that if you make the swaps recommended in this chapter—even just part of the time to start—you will feel and see the benefits. You'll have abounding energy and start to really enjoy nourishing your body with nutritious, anti-inflammatory foods. You'll start eating because you love your body and the way you feel when you eat in an anti-inflammatory way, and you'll start noticing which foods make you feel groggy, irritable, bloated, and sick. If you want to feel energized and flourishing all day, every day— your real, wholesome food intake is the best way to make sure that will happen.

DAILY DETOX THROUGH FOOD

Let's detox, baby! The Maggie Berghoff Way. So long to restrictive and hard detoxes, and hello to the fun, positive, vibrant start to your body reboot! My detox methods are a full detoxification—mind, body, home—to get your life back. It's going to get you feeling, looking, and performing better than you ever have before. It's going to allow you to wipe that white-board clean and start over. No matter what you've tried before, how many doctors you've been to, and how many diets you've been on, this time is different. Take all the confusion, frustration, "to-do" lists, diets, supplements, and recommendations from before and wipe them clean. Start fresh with a bright whiteboard full of endless opportunities. We will decrease your inflammation, boost your immune system, and get your body in a state of optimal health.

Grab a friend or join our community and let's get you feeling amazing daily!

I'm at my best without:

■ **Gluten.** This one is so much easier than it seems. Gluten-free is available at almost every restaurant and store, and almost all my clients have noticed incredible and unintended benefits from nixing gluten. Think: more energy, less brain fog, clearer skin, less bloating . . . one of my clients had dealt with face swelling and a stuffy nose for years, and all of that cleared up when she took out gluten!

■ **Anything heavy in sugars.** Remember, long-term natural sugars are fine . . . in moderation. But added sugars are entirely unnecessary. That's why they're called "added." Your body is far too precious to have icky syrup swimming through your veins. For detox week, we're going to remove even natural sugars like honey, and allow fruit in moderation.

■ **Dairy.** We've learned how dairy can contribute to acne and can be inflammatory. Try to make swaps where you can. Just like gluten, this one is also getting easier by the day. Every coffee shop and restaurant has the option for nut milk or some type of swap-out. You may even like it better.

■ **Anything that makes you feel heavier or more tired.** I'm intentionally vague here because, as I've said repeatedly, everyone's body is so different. You may notice that when you have corn at lunch, you hit an afternoon slump. You may notice that rice in particular bogs you down and deprives you of your creative juices. Or perhaps it's alcohol, and you decide you will no longer partake in alcoholic beverages, or reserve them for only a few special times. Take note of these. It's not always easy to know what's causing your symptoms in regard to food, so you really need to practice homing in on this. That's why when you remove the Triple Trouble items—dairy, grains, sugar—it's SO helpful because it will, as I say, "clear the muddy waters" so you can start to see what's really impacting your health.

Now, let's get excited about what we're bringing MORE of into our lives!

I'm on top of the world with:

- **Leafy vegetables of all colors.** There are so many ways to prepare vegetables simply. Grill them, steam them, eat them raw . . . make a beautiful salad, or a vegetable medley as the perfect complement to a great protein-packed meal. Try out all types of vegetables and get creative about when you eat them, too. For example, having grilled zucchini or peppers with your morning eggs is actually really tasty! Get creative with a morning omelet, or even add some zucchini to your gluten-free muffins.
- **Our anti-inflammatory friends.** Cacao powder, chia seeds, dark chocolate, turmeric, matcha powder, and blueberries are all heaven-sent reprieves for our bodies. It doesn't hurt that they all taste incredible! Add some chia seeds and cacao powder to your morning smoothie, indulge in a chunk of dark chocolate after dinner, treat yourself to a divine matcha latte with almond milk, sprinkle some turmeric into a sauce or a soup on the stove, and snack on a delightful bowl of fresh blueberries. Matcha has less caffeine than coffee so it's gentler on your adrenals, and it has 18 times the antioxidants of blueberries!

For great meal ideas to try with these ingredients, go to chapter 15!

14

YOUR PERSONALIZED DIET RECOMMENDATIONS, PER INFLAMMATION TYPE!

If you're feeling terrible, you want your body to reboot ASAP! Below see my customized advice, per inflammation type! Of course I would love to go into a deep-dive with you on your history, symptoms, and more, but this is going to get you going in the right direction for sure!

MUSCLE AND JOINT INFLAMMATION

What to Eat If You Have Muscle and Joint Inflammation

If you suffer from joint inflammation, add these pain-reducing foods to your grocery list:

- **Bone broth.** It's full of collagen, and great in soup or on its own with some flavoring (like garlic, which is also great for your joints!). My current favorite brand is Bonafide Provisions, and you can find it typically in the freezer section at your grocery store.
- **Vegetables** such as cauliflower, cabbage, broccoli, and onions. As a general rule of thumb, go for color variety in your vegetables.

- **Go for zinc:** pumpkin seeds, oysters, lamb, grass-fed beef, and sesame seeds. Zinc helps with muscle growth and repair. It also helps with nutrient absorption, which in turn will help boost your nutrients, which are needed for healing.
- **Foods with copper** help because copper plays a huge role in collagen production, which helps make bones and tissues. Add avocados, sesame seeds, sunflower seeds, and cashews.
- **Fatty fishes**, like salmon or sardines, which have omega-3 fats, will help decrease inflammation in the body, helping to reduce pain.
- **Nuts** are also high in omega-3 fats and can help greatly in reducing pain and inflammation. Try pistachios, hazelnuts, almonds, and pine nuts.
- **Olive oil** is another great source of omega-3 fat.
- **Tart cherries** are great for joint inflammation. If you suffer from chronic pain syndrome, add tart cherries to your desserts and snack list! They have high levels of antioxidants and anthocyanins, which help to fight inflammation. They've been reported to help lessen pain and soreness. And tart cherry juice is pretty yummy! Grab some to have on hand and drink before you go to sleep, as tart cherries also have naturally occurring melatonin—and, as you know, chronic pain can really make sleep more difficult.
- **Dark chocolate** has antioxidant properties that make it anti-inflammatory! Make sure the chocolate is organic and has a 70 percent cocoa concentration or higher. Yes, I'm giving you the green light for chocolate. I know, right? Being told to eat chocolate? Sign me up! It's all about the quantity and quality of the chocolate.

What Else You Can Do Today to Ease Your Pain

- **Get more sunshine!** Vitamin D may help with inflammation and joint pain, so get outside in the sun at least 15 minutes a day if you can. And you shouldn't wear sunscreen or it will block your ability to synthesize vitamin D. Definitely don't burn, but be sure you have 10–15 minutes in the sun daily before you put on the sunscreen. You may want to consider vitamin D3 plus K2 supplementation year-round as well, as many people are deficient in vitamin D despite outdoor exposure. You want to be sure vitamin K2 is added, as it works together with vitamin D to provide enhanced benefits, especially for bone health, arteries, and your immune system.

- **Check your shoes.** Sometimes, wearing flat shoes like sandals or shoes without arch support can further aggravate the joints within your legs and hips. Don't worry, you don't have to push your favorite pair to the back corner of your closet. There are many great arch-support inserts that can help you while keeping you stylish.

- If you experience joint inflammation in your wrist, thumb, or hands, try a "talk to type" feature when texting or typing on your phone. It will keep your joints from being overused and less likely to inflame.

THREE TOP LIFESTYLE TWEAKS TO TRY FIRST

1. Try an infrared sauna and/or red-light therapy (for more on these, go to page 162).
2. Take an Epsom salt bath three times a week for 30 minutes, or use flotation pods one time a week if possible, once a month minimum. Flotation pods are these massive "pods"

filled with over eleven hundred pounds of Epsom salts. You "float" like you would in the Dead Sea. It's super detoxifying, therapeutic, and healing.

3. Do gentle deep stretching twice daily—right when you wake up, and again in the evening.

HORMONE IMBALANCE

What to Eat to Balance Your Hormones

- **Healthy fats** such as avocados, olive oil, coconut oil, and proteins high in omega-3, like salmon, are important for hormones because of their ability to balance and regulate hormones.
- **Protein.** It's very important to be sure that each of your meals incorporates protein, such as simply prepared chicken, salmon, or turkey. Eggs are also an option if you tolerate them well.
- **Leafy greens and root vegetables.** Get those salads, carrots, beets, and radishes onto your plate! The more color, the better. Spinach in particular is high in iron, which is helpful in balancing hormones.
- **Nuts and seeds** are other great sources of healthy fats. Keep some almonds and pumpkin seeds on hand for snacking. Specifically, try some flax seeds! These small but mighty seeds have phytoestrogen, which can help restore hormonal homeostasis.
- **Sweet potatoes** help with liver detoxification, which can help to stabilize hormones.
- **Sardines** are high in vitamin B12, which can help to balance hormones.

THREE TOP LIFESTYLE TWEAKS TO TRY FIRST

1. Nourish your body as opposed to restricting what you eat. Focus on adding more nutrients and healthy fats. Don't do any sort of restrictive "diet" but rather think, "What can I ADD today to help my body heal itself?"
2. Make sure you take 20 minutes daily of "you time" to brain dump, meditate, stretch, journal, take a walk in nature, or whatever helps you lessen stress. Stress is particularly hard on hormones!
3. Don't work out first thing in the morning on an empty stomach. In fact, you may consider stopping workouts for a period of time as you balance your hormones. Instead, opt for gentle movements such as walking, gentle and enjoyable bike rides, yoga, Pilates, and so forth.

INFLAMMATION FROM SUGAR

What to Eat to Balance Your Blood Sugar

- **Green smoothie.** Start your day with a glass of filtered, high-quality water, followed by a nutrient-dense smoothie. Include healthy fats, protein, greens, and fiber to regulate hormones. You can find recipe tips in the recipe section for smoothies.
- **Swap any "white carbs"** such as pasta, rice, bread, and pastries to better options such as red lentil pasta and almond flour tortillas. Choose gluten-free quinoa or gluten-free rolled oats rather than wheat. In fact, most clients feel best when they avoid grains altogether for at least the time being, so if you're really serious about making some health changes, let's go for grain-free!

THREE TOP LIFESTYLE TWEAKS TO TRY FIRST

1. Move your body (exercise) at least 30 minutes per day. Do something enjoyable to you!
2. Take an Epsom salt bath one to three times a week or try a flotation pod one to four times a month. For more on these, go to page 184.
3. Decrease stress by doing mandatory daily mindset practices. Choose one you know you can stick to consistently! (See chapter 9 for more on mindset.)

INFLAMMATION FROM PSYCHOLOGICAL STRESS

What to Eat If You're Stressed Out

- The following types of **fruits** and **vegetables** are specifically recommended for stress: kiwi, citrus fruits (oranges, lemons, limes), apples, bananas, cucumbers, grapefruit, spinach, and carrots.
- **Leafy greens** and a wide variety of vegetables support brain function!
- **Healthy fats** such as avocados, nut butters, and salmon also supercharge your mind.

What Else You Can Do Today to Lighten Your Mood

- **Get creative** when you feel stress coming on. This could include scrapbooking, journaling, painting—whatever you can do to get into a creative flow.
- **Call on your best pal, endorphins!** Get some exercise, it usually helps. It may also help to exercise in workout classes or in a group—human connection is so helpful for combating mental and psychological stress, even when

you feel like you don't want it. Try to avoid frequent alcohol use, at least for the time being. I love a good martini as much as the next person, but alcohol can further interfere with your brain and emotions, making it challenging to strike a balance.

■ Anything that can bring you out of the sympathetic nervous system is ideal for coping with anxiety. Many prefer **meditation** and **yoga**: practices that focus on slowing the breath, which decreases heart rate and signals to the body that everything is OK. Try some breathing exercises and slow and easy stretches.

THREE TOP LIFESTYLE TWEAKS TO TRY FIRST

1. Get outside every single morning to see the sun and breathe fresh air.
2. Heal your gut. Most neurotransmitters are made in your gut, so improving gut health will help improve mental health. Take your gut-healing supplementations daily.
3. Try yoga or some other stretching exercise while playing soft music.

INFLAMMATION FROM DIGESTIVE STRESS

What to Eat to Calm Your Stomach

■ **Ginger.** Ginger is widely beloved for settling the digestive tract when things don't feel great. It can also reduce bloating. Try ginger tea, or use ginger when cooking.

■ **Foods with probiotics**, such as kimchi, sauerkraut, and Bubbies brand pickles. These probiotics will work to rebalance the gut microbiota. You can also take a probiotic pill.

- **Apple cider vinegar** with the "mother" in it (this refers to the brown stuff that floats around at the bottom) is also exceptional for digestive help. You can add 1–2 tablespoons into some warm water with freshly squeezed lemon juice and a dash of cinnamon to help with digestion and detoxification!
- **Leafy greens.** Go for a variety—spinach, cabbage, kale, arugula.
- **Foods that are high in fiber,** such as chia seeds, apples, and fennel.

Foods That Help Ease Constipation

- **Prunes** or prune juice
- **Fruits** such as pears, apples, kiwi, and citrus fruits (lemons, limes, and oranges)
- **Leafy greens** like spinach
- **A morning smoothie** and green juice to get things moving
- **Lemon water**

Foods That Help Stop Diarrhea

- In a severe situation, it's common to want bread, rice, and bananas to help soothe diarrhea. However, these foods ironically are often the very things making your gut inflammation WORSE. Instead, focus on the bigger goal—to eliminate the diarrhea for good. Think, "What can I ADD to totally heal and nourish my body?" Imagine your gut lining soaking in all the nutrients and vibrant colors. Imagine your immune system getting stronger with every sip or bite. Is rice going to do that? NO! Choose vegetables. And, I know that vegetables are the last thing you want right now when struggling with diarrhea, so sneak them in instead. Remember, the goal is to rebalance the gut for good and change the entire internal environment.

▪ A great way to sneak **veggies** in: make some gluten-free zucchini bread muffins to have on hand. Be sure you're stocked up with frozen greens to make a big creamy smoothie packed with greens and antioxidants. Try overnight oats for that soothing "carb" feel but add coconut oil, chia seeds, collagen powder, and nut butter to make it delicious, easy, fast, AND great for rebalancing your gut. I mention these items because you never know when you're going to have a super-bad "diarrhea" day, and you want to have these on hand. You can prep them ahead of time and even keep the zucchini muffins in the freezer.

How to Ease Bloating

▪ The above foods, for sure, but in an acute situation my favorite hack is **rubbing peppermint oil on the belly**. I recommend using it before bedtime under your PJs, or even during the day if you're just lounging around at home. It's a lifesaver.

▪ **A LOT of water.** Water will help debloat significantly.

▪ **Squeeze lemon into your water** and add a dash of cayenne pepper if you dare. This is amazing for reducing bloating and detoxification.

THREE TOP LIFESTYLE TWEAKS TO TRY FIRST

1. Do a daily mindset and relaxation exercise to get into your parasympathetic nervous state and out of your

sympathetic nervous state (for more on mindset, go to page 132). Focus on balanced breathing prior to eating anything.

2. Chew your food until it's liquid, and eat slowly. Eating quickly and failing to chew all the way can cause problems. Yes, this means I want you to take a real meal break . . . no more downing your breakfast while walking into work, eating lunch while simultaneously typing on your computer or getting through more emails, and eating dinner while watching TV. Take a break and truly think about the meal you're eating. A lot of times we eat so quickly and absentmindedly that all of a sudden it's gone and we almost "blacked out" during it all! Not OK. Sit down, look at the colors of your food, appreciate the nourishment you're about to put in your body, think about your cells becoming charged and fulfilled with every bite, chew and imagine your food filling up your energy reserves so you can become a more powerful and vibrant person.

3. Take targeted supplements for digestion, healing the gut lining, and healthy bowel movements to help bridge the gap between your current digestive distress and healing for good.

ALLERGY, ASTHMA, AND SKIN INFLAMMATION

What to Eat to Support Your Respiratory System and Your Skin

- **Foods high in vitamin D**, such as fatty fishes (salmon) and whole eggs.
- **Nuts and seeds.** These are high in vitamin E, which has tocopherol, which has been shown to help with coughing and asthma! One of my favorite things to do is fill a bag

with nuts and seeds at a local whole-foods store, and have it for snacking throughout the week. I keep mine in the freezer—try it, it's so good.

■ **Vegetables**, such as leafy greens and carrots.

THREE TOP LIFESTYLE TWEAKS TO TRY FIRST

1. Get a high-quality air filtration system in your home, and do a deep clean.
2. Use only nontoxic, organic, unscented beauty, household, and hygiene products.
3. Hydrate fully. Be sure to drink high-quality water and a minimum of 8–10 glasses a day.

15

MAGGIE BERGHOFF'S
BODY RESET

Ready for an MBBR (Maggie Berghoff's Body Reset)? Now is the time to commit to and implement a new beginning. This is a time to reduce things that may be causing inflammation, and add things that will fuel you to be your greatest. When initially making these changes, you may feel cravings, headaches, sleepy, or even a bit nauseated. Give yourself some grace and really spend time relaxing in nature, pampering yourself, journaling, and envisioning your best self. Drink a lot of water to flush out toxins and consider adding things such as flotation therapy and massage in order to help get rid of the toxins and reset your body. You can also get in an infrared sauna, which is a sauna that also provides infrared therapy to detoxify, relieve pain, improve circulation, and so much more. I've included some recipes here to help you in your reset with ideas of what to make that will automatically be anti-inflammatory and detoxifying! Stick to the concepts of anti-inflammatory choices in general long-term, but without being restrictive or fearful of food choices. Simply focus on general everyday wellness, a healthy mindset and nourishing diet, and prioritizing your health!

The following are some guidelines that will help reset your body and rewire yourself to be stronger, healthier, and happier:

DAILY

- No grains
- No sugar
- No dairy
- Minimum 5 servings of vegetables; aim to really boost your veggie intake
- 1 gallon of water
- 30 minutes of movement
- Take targeted supplements specific to your body's needs
- Follow all of the grocery/pantry ingredient recommendations (e.g., no inflammatory oils, limit fruits, etc.)
- Choose one thing we outlined in the Mindset and Mindfulness chapter to implement to your life each day

WEEKLY

- Take an Epsom salt bath or go to a flotation tank session

EXTRAS

Here are some ideas you may want to "add on" to your Body Reset. This is YOUR body and your life. Some of my clients remove the standards from their daily nutrition (e.g., gluten, sugar), and some—especially my elite athletes and CEOs— always go the extra mile. You get to choose your path and how you go through each day:

- No alcohol
- No caffeine
- Meditation
- Yoga
- Outdoors every morning
- Dry brushing
- Red-light therapy
- Infrared sauna
- One serving of fruit a day only
- No eating past 6:30 p.m.
- In bed by 9:30 p.m.
- Journaling
- Read daily
- No social media/phones/devices past 7:00 p.m.
- Switch household items to nontoxic choices
- Switch makeup, bathroom, shower items to nontoxic choices
- Massage/facials

ANTI-INFLAMMATORY RECIPES

Here you'll find some go-to recipes for anti-inflammatory living. Investing in nontoxic cookware and an Instant Pot will be helpful. Also, I've noted some dietary specifications above each recipe to help target your needs. We have not gone into detail on "nightshades—" but these are foods such as potatoes, eggplant, and tomatoes that may cause increased inflammation in some people. You may consider removing them for a period of time based on the severity of your health concerns.

Key:
GF – Gluten-Free
GRF – Grain-Free
DF – Dairy-Free
SF – Sugar-Free
NSF – Nightshade-Free
EF – Egg-Free

I hope you enjoy these as much as we do!!

Note: Only cook/bake with the approved oils listed in chapter 13, avoiding oils such as canola, cottonseed, and peanut.

ALMOND FLOUR "OATMEAL"

GF – GRF – DF – SF – NSF – EF

Prep time: 2 minutes ■ Cook time: 8 minutes ■ Total time: 10 minutes

This grain-free porridge has all the comforting creaminess of a warm bowl of oatmeal with anti-inflammatory benefits from almond flour, turmeric, and ginger. It's the perfect balance of spice and warmth for a chilly morning.   *Serves: 1*

3 tablespoons almond flour
2 tablespoons flax meal
½ teaspoon vanilla extract
¼ teaspoon ground turmeric
Pinch of ground ginger
½ cup unsweetened almond milk or other dairy-free milk
2 to 3 drops liquid stevia, or to taste
Pinch of salt

In a small saucepan, stir together the almond flour, flax meal, vanilla, turmeric, ginger, milk, sweetener, and salt. Bring to a simmer, reduce the heat to low, and cook for 5 minutes, stirring regularly, until thick and creamy. Add more milk for a thinner consistency if you like.

PUMPKIN PIE CHIA PUDDING

GF – GRF – DF – SF – NSF – EF

Prep time: 1 hour ■ Total time: 1 hour

I love the seasonal flavor of this vitamin A–packed breakfast. You can prep a big batch over the weekend to keep in the fridge and enjoy creamy chia pudding for breakfast all week long.

Serves: 1

4 tablespoons chia seeds
1 cup unsweetened almond or coconut milk
¼ cup pumpkin puree
¼ cup unsweetened plain dairy-free yogurt
¼ teaspoon vanilla extract
½ teaspoon ground cinnamon or pumpkin pie spice
Pinch of salt
Optional toppings: nut butter, coconut flakes, cacao bits

1. In a container with a lid, whisk together the chia seeds, milk, pumpkin, yogurt, vanilla, cinnamon, and salt until smooth.
2. Cover the container and refrigerate for at least 1 hour and up to overnight. Add toppings, if using, and enjoy!

BREAKFAST

VEGGIE SCRAMBLE

GF – GRF – DF – SF – NSF

Prep time: 5 minutes ■ Cook time: 7 minutes ■ Total time: 12 minutes

This is my favorite way to start the day—with tons of vegetables and protein. I don't always feel like it, but it's worth it to get those nutrients in your body right away! You can use any combination of colorful vegetables you have on hand to maximize morning nutrition. *Serves: 1*

> 1 teaspoon coconut oil
> 1 garlic clove, minced
> 1 cup fresh baby spinach, coarsely chopped
> 2 large eggs, beaten (can substitute crumbled tofu for
>   egg-free)
> Salt and pepper
> Grain-free tortilla
> Fresh basil, for garnish

1. In a large skillet, heat the oil over medium heat. Add the garlic and cook for 1 to 2 minutes. Add the spinach and cook until wilted, 1 to 2 minutes.
2. Pour in the eggs and gently stir into the veggies until just set. Season to taste with salt and pepper.
3. Transfer the scramble to a tortilla and garnish with basil to serve.

LUNCH

CURRIED CHICKPEA SALAD WRAPS

GF – GRF – DF – SF – NSF – EF

Prep time: 7 minutes ■ Total time: 7 minutes

This vegan lunch recipe is just as creamy and savory as your favorite chicken salad, with an anti-inflammatory boost (and sunny color!) from the turmeric in curry powder. *Serves: 2*

½ cup unsweetened plain dairy-free yogurt (almond or
    coconut)
½ lemon, juiced
1 to 2 teaspoons curry powder, or to taste
½ teaspoon garlic powder
½ teaspoon salt, or to taste
¼ teaspoon black pepper
1 (15-ounce) can chickpeas, rinsed and drained
2 celery stalks, diced
1 scallion, minced
2 grain-free wraps
2 cups baby arugula

1. In a medium bowl, whisk together the yogurt, lemon juice, curry powder, garlic powder, salt, and pepper until smooth. Taste and adjust the seasoning with salt, pepper, and/or lemon juice.
2. Fold in the chickpeas, celery, and scallion until fully combined.
3. Lay the wraps on a work surface and place a layer of arugula in the center of each wrap. Divide the chickpea salad between the wraps and fold to close.

LEMON-SPINACH EGG DROP SOUP

GF – GRF – DF – SF – NSF

Prep time: 5 minutes ■ Cook time: 15 minutes ■ Total time: 20 minutes

This vibrant soup comes together quickly and is packed with gut health benefits from bone broth and a bright, sunny flavor from freshly squeezed lemon juice.   *Serves: 4*

> *1 teaspoon coconut oil*
> *2 garlic cloves, minced*
> *3 scallions, minced, white and green parts separated*
> *8 cups chicken bone broth*
> *4 cups fresh baby spinach*
> *4 large eggs, lightly beaten*
> *1 lemon, juiced*
> *Himalayan salt*

1. Heat the oil in a stockpot over medium heat until melted. Add the garlic and scallion whites and sauté until fragrant, about 1 minute.
2. Add the broth and bring to a simmer.
3. Reduce the heat to maintain a simmer (not a boil). Add the spinach and cook until wilted, about 2 minutes.
4. With the soup at a simmer, slowly pour the beaten eggs into the soup while continuously whisking in a counterclockwise direction to make ribbons with the eggs. Stir for about 2 minutes, until the eggs are just set, then remove from the heat.
5. Add the lemon juice and season with salt. Serve with the remaining scallion greens for garnish.

COBB SALAD

GF – GRF – DF – SF – NSF

Prep time: 10 minutes ■ Cook time: 5 minutes ■ Total time: 15 minutes

It's time to bring this classic salad into a new light with a creamy dairy-free herby dressing, crisp turkey bacon, and peppery arugula. This is an absolute staple in my home—and I always keep a big premade portion in the fridge to dish out throughout the week. Just be sure to keep the dressing separate and mix it in just before you're going to eat it. PS: This is hubby-approved! And he typically is NOT a salad kinda guy.   *Serves: 2*

Dressing
½ cup raw cashews, soaked
    in boiling water for at
    least 15 minutes
¼ cup fresh dill fronds
¼ cup chopped fresh chives
½ lemon, juiced
Pinch of pink Himalayan
    salt

Salad
6 slices turkey bacon
5 ounces arugula
1 English cucumber,
    peeled and sliced
2 hard-boiled eggs, sliced
    (omit for egg-free)

1. Drain the cashews and place in a blender, along with the dill, chives, lemon juice, and salt. Blend until smooth, adding water, 1 tablespoon at a time, to reach a pourable consistency. Season to taste.
2. Heat a large skillet over medium heat and cook the bacon until crisp. Transfer to a paper towel–lined plate to cool. Once cool, crumble the bacon.
3. In a large bowl, toss the arugula and cucumber with the dressing. Divide between serving bowls and top with crumbled bacon and eggs.

DINNER

SHRIMP CAULIFLOWER FRIED RICE

GF – GRF – DF – SF – NSF – EF

Prep time: 5 minutes ■ Cook time: 15 minutes ■ Total time: 20 minutes

You won't miss the grains in this all-vegetable, soy-free fried rice. This recipe is full of flavor, protein, and vegetables, but it won't weigh you down like your typical take-out order. It's SO good—you must make this . . . trust me on this one!　*Serves: 4*

2 tablespoons coconut oil
1 pound large shrimp, peeled and deveined
Salt and black pepper
1 tablespoon minced fresh ginger
2 garlic cloves, minced
4 scallions, minced, white and green parts separated
2 large carrots, cut into thin rounds
1 zucchini, diced
16 ounces riced cauliflower, or 1 small head cauliflower
　　broken down into florets and riced in a food processor
3 cups chopped kale
2 tablespoons coconut aminos

1. In a large skillet or wok, melt 1 tablespoon of the oil over medium heat. Add the shrimp and sprinkle with salt and pepper. Cook for 2 to 3 minutes, flipping halfway through, until the shrimp is pink and curled into a "C" shape. Transfer the shrimp to a plate and cover to keep warm.

2. Melt the remaining 1 tablespoon oil over medium heat. Add the ginger, garlic, and scallion whites and sauté for 1 minute. Add the carrots and zucchini and cook for 5 minutes, until softened.

3. Add the cauliflower rice and kale and cook until heated through and the kale is wilted. Stir in the shrimp and coconut aminos. Divide among plates and garnish with scallion greens to serve.

DINNER

SEARED SALMON WITH LIME-AVOCADO SALSA
GF – GRF – DF – SF – NSF – EF

Prep time: 35 minutes ■ Cook time: 15 minutes ■ Total time: 50 minutes

Omega-3-rich salmon gets a zesty and bright dressing from a fast lime-avocado salsa. This low-sugar salsa is just as tasty on salmon as it is on veggie tacos or your morning eggs.

Serves: 4

Salmon
- 1 teaspoon salt
- 1 teaspoon smoked paprika
- 1 teaspoon ground cumin
- ½ teaspoon ground turmeric
- 4 (6- to 8-ounce) salmon fillets
- 1 lemon, sliced into thin rounds

Salsa
- 1 avocado, diced
- ¼ red onion, diced
- ⅓ cup coarsely chopped cilantro
- 1 to 2 limes, juiced
- Salt

1. In a small bowl, combine the 1 teaspoon salt, the paprika, cumin, and turmeric. Coat the salmon in the spice mixture, cover, and refrigerate for 30 minutes to 4 hours.
2. Preheat the oven to 450°F. Line a baking sheet with parchment paper.
3. Place the salmon on the prepared baking sheet. Cover each fillet with 2 to 3 slices of lemon. Roast for 12 to 15 minutes, until the salmon is cooked through.
4. Meanwhile, combine the avocado, onion, cilantro, and lime juice in a medium bowl. Season with salt.
5. Serve the salmon with salsa.

CHICKEN AND VEGETABLE SHEET PAN DINNER

GF – GRF – DF – SF – NSF – EF

Prep time: 5 minutes ■ Cook time: 30 minutes ■ Total time: 35 minutes

You only need one sheet pan to whip up this fast and healthy weeknight dinner. It's family-friendly and easy to customize using any vegetables you have on hand. Mix it up a little each time!   *Serves: 4*

2 small sweet potatoes, cut into 1-inch pieces
1 teaspoon salt, plus more to taste
Black pepper
2 large chicken breasts, cut into 1-inch pieces
2 small heads broccoli, cut into florets
1 yellow squash, cut into ½-inch half-moons
1 lemon, juiced
1 tablespoon Italian seasoning
1 teaspoon onion powder
1 teaspoon ground turmeric

1. Preheat the oven to 400°F. Line a baking sheet with parchment paper.
2. On the prepared baking sheet, toss the sweet potatoes with a generous pinch of salt and pepper. Roast for 10 minutes while you prepare the remaining ingredients (the potatoes take a bit longer to cook).
3. Meanwhile, in a large bowl, toss the chicken, broccoli, squash, lemon juice, Italian seasoning, onion powder, turmeric, and the 1 teaspoon salt.
4. When the sweet potatoes have roasted for 10 minutes, remove the baking sheet from the oven and add the chicken and vegetables to the baking sheet. Spread into an even layer.
5. Roast for 15 to 20 minutes, stirring after 7 minutes. The chicken is done when it's no longer pink in the center.

DINNER

INSTANT POT PULLED CHICKEN

GF – GRF – DF – SF – NSF – EF

Prep time: 2 minutes ■ Cook time: 30 minutes ■ Total time: 32 minutes

You'll be amazed by how just four ingredients (plus salt and black pepper) turn into a saucy and thick pulled chicken recipe. Enjoy it hot out of the Instant Pot, make quick chicken tacos, or top a salad with chilled chicken for lunch the next day. This is my personal favorite go-to. I keep Instant Pot chicken in the fridge for easy shredding onto a salad or with veggies when I need a quick meal!   *Serves: 4*

3 boneless, skinless chicken breasts
½ cup coconut aminos
½ cup bone broth
2 tablespoons chia seeds
Salt and black pepper

1. Place the chicken, coconut aminos, and broth in an Instant Pot (or pressure cooker). Lock the lid in place and select High Pressure for 10 minutes. When the timer beeps, turn off the Instant Pot and let the pressure release naturally for 5 minutes, then finish with a quick pressure release.
2. When all the steam is let out, carefully remove the lid using a hot pad. Stir in the chia seeds and let the mixture sit for 5 minutes to thicken up. Shred the meat and season to taste.
3. Store in an airtight container for up to 5 days. Serve with veggies, in an almond flour wrap, with avocado, or with a stir-fry.

ANTI-INFLAMMATORY TRUFFLES

GF – GRF – DF – SF – NSF – EF

Prep time: 10 minutes ■ Total time: 10 minutes

I'm a HUGE fan of dark chocolate—like, huge. Indulge in these decadent, chocolate and cinnamon refrigerator truffles that happen to be refined sugar–free (it's amazing what a couple of dates can do!).   *Makes: 12*

> 2 Medjool dates, soaked in hot water for 10 minutes and
>   drained
> ¾ cup unsweetened creamy almond butter
> ⅔ cup hemp seeds
> 3 tablespoons unsweetened cocoa powder
> 1 teaspoon ground cinnamon
> 3 tablespoons chia seeds
> Pinch of salt
> ½ teaspoon vanilla extract

1. In a food processor, blend the dates and almond butter into a paste.
2. Add the hemp seeds, cocoa powder, cinnamon, chia seeds, salt, and vanilla, and blend until you have a cohesive dough.
3. Roll the dough into 12 balls. If you like, roll the balls in cocoa powder to coat. Store in an airtight container in the fridge for up to 2 weeks, or in the freezer for up to 3 months.

SWEET POTATO TOAST

GF – GRF – DF – SF – NSF – EF

Prep time: 2 minutes ■ Cook time: 10 minutes ■ Total time: 12 minutes

love to turn sweet potatoes, a fantastic source of vitamin A, into cute, naturally sweet toast slices! Garnish each slice with any of your favorite sweet or savory toppings and enjoy!

Serves: 2

1 large sweet potato, sliced into ¼-inch planks
Topping suggestions: mashed avocado, sliced tomato, nut
    butter, dairy-free yogurt, dried seasonings, ground
    cinnamon, ground turmeric, hot sauce

1. Preheat the oven to 400°F.
2. Place the sweet potato slices on a baking sheet and roast for 10 minutes. Flip and roast for another 10 to 15 minutes, until cooked through.
3. Let the sweet potato cool slightly and top with the toppings of your choice.

VEGGIE EGG MUFFINS

GF – GRF – DF – SF – NSF

Prep time: 10 minutes ■ Cook time: 25 minutes ■ Total time: 35 minutes

These vegetable-packed egg muffins make an ideal on-the-go breakfast or afternoon pick-me-up. Plus, they're fully kid-approved! I've actually found anything in muffin shape is more likely to be kid-approved—try it out!   *Serves: 12*

> *12 large eggs*
> *1 teaspoon salt*
> *½ white onion, diced*
> *1 medium yellow squash, diced*

1. Preheat the oven to 350°F. Lightly grease a 12-cup muffin tin with coconut or avocado oil spray.
2. In a large bowl, whisk the eggs and salt until totally smooth.
3. Divide the onion and yellow squash among the muffin cups.
4. Pour the whisked eggs into the muffin cups. Pick the tin up and gently tap it on the counter a few times to settle the eggs.
5. Place the muffin tin on a baking sheet (to catch any overflow) and bake for 20 to 25 minutes, until the centers are set.
6. Let the muffins cool for 5 to 10 minutes in the muffin tin before removing them from the tin. Store the muffins in the fridge for up to 5 days, or freeze for up to 3 months.

DESSERT/SNACKS

ZUCCHINI MUFFINS
GF – GRF – DF – SF – NSF

Prep time: 10 minutes ■ Cook time: 25 minutes ■ Total time: 35 minutes

Coconut flour and collagen protein powder make the fluffiest grain-free zucchini muffins with benefits. Plus, fresh zucchini keeps the muffins perfectly moist for breakfast or a not-too-sweet after-dinner treat.   *Makes: 12*

⅔ cup coconut flour
½ cup coconut sugar
¼ cup collagen protein powder
2 teaspoons baking powder
1 teaspoon ground cinnamon
½ teaspoon ground ginger
¼ teaspoon salt
2 cups shredded zucchini, squeezed dry in a dish cloth
6 large eggs
¼ cup melted coconut oil, cooled
3 tablespoons water
*Optional: ½ cup chopped walnuts or dairy-free chocolate
    chips*

1. Preheat the oven to 350°F and line a 12-cup muffin tin with paper liners.
2. In a large bowl, whisk together the coconut flour, sugar, collagen, baking powder, cinnamon, ginger, and salt. Add the zucchini, eggs, oil, and water. Add another tablespoon of water if the batter is very thick. It should be scoopable, not as thin and pourable as regular muffin batter.
3. Fold in the nuts and/or chocolate chips, if using.
4. Divide the batter among the prepared muffin cups and bake for 25 minutes, until golden brown and firm to the touch.
5. Cool the muffins in the muffin tin.

DRINKS

ICED MATCHA LATTE

GF – GRF – DF – SF – NSF – EF

Prep time: 3 minutes ■ Total time: 3 minutes

'm a huge fan of creamy iced matcha lattes, and make them often! I don't like matcha tea plain, so if you're the same—try this recipe! This potent powdered green tea has just the right amount of caffeine to perk you up without the jitters, and is overflowing with antioxidants.   *Serves: 1*

> *½ to 1 teaspoon matcha tea*
> *1 serving collagen peptides*
> *1 cup unsweetened almond milk*
> *Liquid stevia, to taste*

1. Put the matcha tea, collagen peptides, milk, and stevia in a blender and blend on high until smooth. Alternatively, you can use an immersion blender or a frother.
2. Pour over ice to serve.

COLLAGEN COFFEE LATTE

GF – GRF – DF – SF – NSF – EF

Prep time: 5 minutes ■ Total time: 5 minutes

Drink the gut-healing benefits of collagen in your coffee! This creamy blended latte drink is an easy way to add extra protein to your morning. Add ice for more of a shake-like texture.   *Serves: 1*

6 ounces brewed coffee
1 scoop collagen peptides
2 tablespoons dairy-free milk
Liquid stevia, to taste

1. Put the brewed coffee, collagen peptides, milk, and stevia in a blender and blend on high until smooth. Alternatively, you can use an immersion blender or a frother.
2. Pour over ice to serve.

DRINKS

BERRIES AND GREENS SMOOTHIE

GF – GRF – DF – SF – NSF – EF

Prep time: 5 minutes ■ Total time: 5 minutes

Frozen berries add just the right amount of sweetness to balance the spinach in this antioxidant-packed smoothie.

Serves: 1

1 cup frozen raspberries, blueberries, and/or strawberries
1 serving collagen peptides or plant protein powder
½ teaspoon ground cinnamon
2 handfuls fresh baby spinach
1 cup unsweetened almond butter
4 ice cubes

Put the berries, collagen peptides, cinnamon, spinach, almond butter, and ice in a blender and blend until smooth.

DRINKS

ALMOND BUTTER CUP SMOOTHIE

GF – GRF – DF – SF – NSF – EF

Prep time: 5 minutes ■ Total time: 5 minutes

This creamy smoothie tastes like dessert for breakfast! Who doesn't want to start their day with peanut butter and chocolate? I always add a scoop of collagen peptides for extra protein, too!   *Serves: 1*

1 tablespoon unsweetened almond butter
1 teaspoon unsweetened cocoa powder
1 handful fresh baby spinach
1½ cups unsweetened almond milk
1 serving collagen peptides or plant protein powder

Put the almond butter, cocoa powder, spinach, milk, and collagen peptides in a blender and blend until smooth.

DRINKS

GREEN PROTEIN SMOOTHIE

GF – GRF – DF – SF – NSF – EF

Prep time: 5 minutes ■ Total time: 5 minutes

Avocado is the secret to an incredibly fluffy and creamy smoothie. You don't need much else to make this protein-rich smoothie that is guaranteed to hold you over until lunch.

Serves: 1

½ *small ripe avocado*
1 *serving collagen peptides or plant-based protein powder*
2 *generous handfuls fresh baby spinach*
1½ *cups unsweetened almond milk or coconut water*
Optional: ½ *teaspoon cinnamon, turmeric, lemon juice,*
   fresh mint

Place the avocado, collagen peptides, spinach, and milk in a blender and blend until smooth. Add 4 to 5 ice cubes instead of ½ cup of the liquid for a thicker consistency.

GREEN JUICE

GF – GRF – DF – SF – NSF – EF

Prep time: 10 minutes ■ Total time: 10 minutes

Make your own refreshing and thirst-quenching green juice with your favorite leafy greens, celery, cucumber, and parsley. Ginger adds a gentle spicy flavor and digestive benefits. Yes, it takes extra time to make your own juices, but if you can make it a habit, I think you'll find it enjoyable! *Serves: 2*

1 bunch kale
1-inch-piece fresh ginger, peeled
5 celery stalks
1 English cucumber
½ bunch fresh parsley

1. Coarsely chop all the ingredients.
2. Put the kale, ginger, celery, cucumber, and parsley in a juicer. Alternatively, add them to a blender and blend on high, then strain the juice through a fine-mesh strainer.

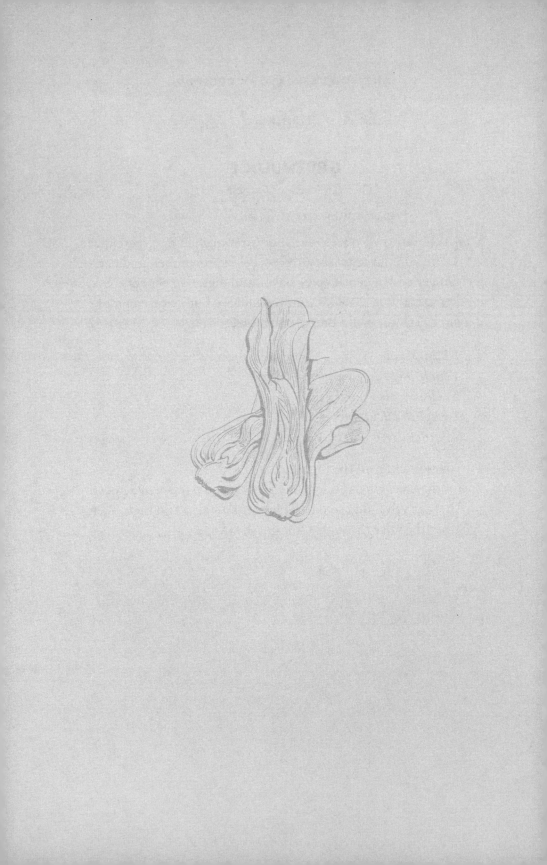

TO LESS STRESS . . .
AND A HAPPY LIFE!

We went through a lot together in this book. First, THANK YOU for trusting me and allowing me to help you on this journey. I am forever honored and humbled to be in a position to help spread health and wellness your way. I also would love to connect with you and hear about your health journey and things you are implementing from this book, so feel free to reach out to me any time on social media or via my website. Second, I want you to know and believe that you CAN heal your body when you make specific lifestyle changes and eat to treat. A vibrant, energetic, and adventurous life awaits you. Every day just do one next step that will nourish your mind, body, and soul, and that will lead you to the anti-inflammatory and symptom-free lifestyle you deserve. I'm so excited for your transformation, and for you to truly redesign yourself! You can do this!

With love,

Maggie Berghoff

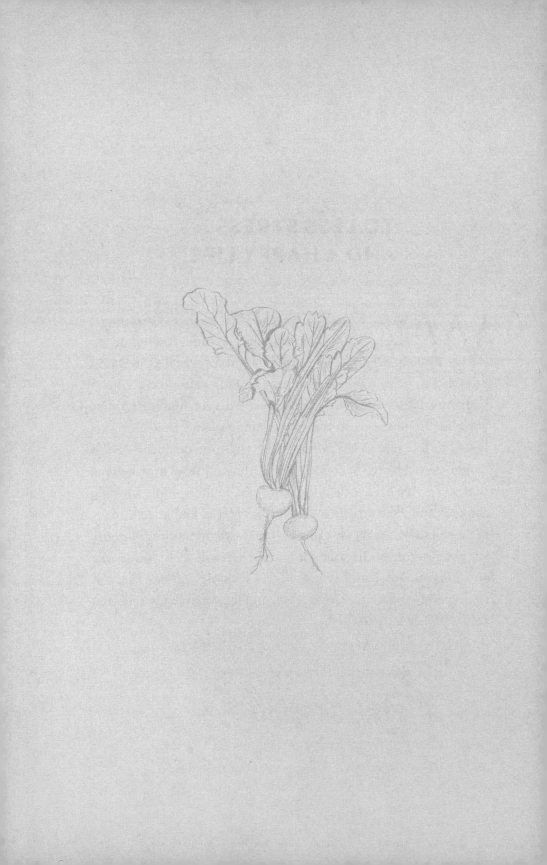

IDENTIFY YOUR
INFLAMMATION TYPE QUIZ

Please rate the below symptoms on a scale of 0–3.

    0 – Not present

    1 – Present a few days a month

    2 – Present a few weeks a month

    3 – Present almost always

MUSCLE AND JOINT INFLAMMATION

_____ I experience physical pain in my muscles.

_____ I experience physical pain in my joints.

_____ I get shooting pains down my arms and legs, or numbness and tingling in my hands or feet.

_____ I wake up stiff or have stiffness throughout the day.

_____ My joints are warm or hot to the touch, or even appear red at times.

CATEGORY TOTAL: _____

HORMONAL INFLAMMATION AND THE THYROID

_____ The outer thirds of my eyebrows are thin or missing, and/or my hair is thinning.

_____ My body swells up at times or I am gaining weight. I notice my rings fitting tighter, my face "puffy," or my legs swollen toward the bottom especially.

_____ For energy, one (or all) of these apply to me:

- I wake up tired even if I get eight-plus hours of sleep.
- I crash in the middle of the afternoon and sometimes get a "second wind" late in the evening.
- By about 3 p.m. I am so tired and drained for the rest of the day. I have no energy in the evening at all.

_____ I'm cold all the time.

_____ My cycles are irregular or nonexistent.

CATEGORY TOTAL: _____

INFLAMMATION CAUSED BY SUGAR

_____ I feel lightheaded/dizzy/shaky/irritable.

_____ I rarely seem to feel full and satisfied, and crave carbs and sugars often.

_____ I'm excessively thirsty.

_____ I've been gaining weight, or can't lose weight.

_____ I have excess fat around my abdomen, sides, or back.

CATEGORY TOTAL: _____

PSYCHOLOGICAL STRESS

_____ I experience anxiety and/or at times feel like my heart is racing.

_____ I'm often unmotivated. I've lost joy for things I used to love.

_____ I feel forgetful or have brain fog. I can't remember things, I lose things, and I often miss things.

_____ My mood is irritable often.

_____ My mood fluctuates; sometimes I'm super happy and other times I'm very sad.

CATEGORY TOTAL: _____

DIGESTIVE INFLAMMATION

_____ I have constipation or diarrhea.

_____ I feel like I "look pregnant," no matter what I eat, and am bloated often.

_____ I get heartburn or acid reflux after eating or if I haven't eaten in a while.

_____ When I eat food, I experience some sort of symptom, which could include feeling tired, in pain, breaking out, or moody.

_____ After I eat, I'm still hungry.

CATEGORY TOTAL: _____

ALLERGIES, ASTHMA, AND SKIN INFLAMMATION

_____ I have excessively dry or oily skin.

_____ My skin is typically red, inflamed, patchy, or itchy and/or I have unexplained rashes.

_____ I feel like my head is a balloon.

_____ It feels hard to get a full breath, like my lungs aren't working fully.

_____ I hear a wheezing sound when I breathe in/out.

_____ My eyes are red, swollen, itchy, or puffy.

CATEGORY TOTAL: _____

RESULTS

Thank you for filling out the Identify Your Inflammation Type Quiz. This assessment gives you an idea of the type of inflammation you are dealing with, and it can give you insight into where to start with your health journey, as well as what to tell your doctor you suspect in regards to your symptoms.

Below is a scale indicating the level of severity to which the inflammation you are experiencing would fall, in EACH category. Take your score and match it up within the ranges provided. This is not to be taken as a cumulative score, but rather an individual score within each inflammation category above. This will tell you where to focus your efforts first and second, depending on where your highest inflammatory levels appear.

Severity	Score Range
Level 1	0–5
Level 2	6–10
Level 3	11–15
Level 4	16–20

LEVEL 1: 0 → 5

Symptoms do not typically interfere with your daily activities. Some days, you feel amazing and don't notice any symptoms at all. However, trouble may be lurking, and there may be imbalances in your body chemistry that, if we do not address them right now, may cause problems later. Implement a few fine-tuning changes that will prevent decline and help you feel even better!

LEVEL 2: 6 → 10

At this level of inflammation, you're likely starting to notice you just aren't the same as you used to be. You may be blaming it on work, stress, aging, or diet, but the truth is—you have some imbalances in your body chemistry that are catching up to you. It's only a matter of time before one more "hit" comes at you, and your body can no longer compensate and you'll start to experience major burnout, symptoms, and even autoimmune disease. I recommend that you have a comprehensive case review with a functional medicine practitioner where you will be given the laboratory work needed to ensure customized strategies going forward to stop this inflammation.

LEVEL 3: 11 → 15

You're definitely feeling poorly, and I'm sending you so much love. Tired, gut issues, skin not looking the same as it once did, motivation dropping, body physique struggling, aches and pains. You've likely tried some things to feel better—maybe a supplement that promised a magic fix, a diet program, or a detox. Time to find out exactly what is causing this inflammation, and how to reverse it, so you know what to do step-by-step to get fully better.

LEVEL 4: 16 → 20

You may feel hopeless, frustrated, and honestly about to just give up and accept this is your life. However, I want you to know there IS hope. I know you've bounced around to so many doctor's appointments. I know you've tried so many things and are still feeling horrible. I know this has impacted not even just you, but those around you as well. Your biggest task right now is to get your mindset right, believe with everything in you that you CAN and WILL heal, or at least greatly reduce your symptoms and lead a higher quality of life. Do small things, day by day, and just keep putting one foot in front of the other. If you are able to, find a great functional medicine practitioner to hold your hand through this, get to the root cause of your illness, and lead you to your best self.

TOTAL TOXIC BURDEN QUIZ

Rate each of the following based on your last 30 days.

Point Scale:

    0 = Never or almost never

    1 = Occasionally have it, symptom is not severe

    2 = Occasionally have it, symptom is severe

    3 = Frequently have it, symptom is not severe

    4 = Frequently have it, symptom is severe

Please note that this total number may be fairly high when you first complete this quiz. That is quite common. Your number today is a starting point, and by implementing the strategies within this book, your number will begin to decrease over time.

HEAD

____ Headaches

____ Migraines

____ Dizzinesss

                       CATEGORY TOTAL: _____

SLEEP

____ Can't fall asleep

____ Fall asleep but wake up in the middle of the night

____ Wake up still tired even after sleeping

                       CATEGORY TOTAL: _____

EYES

____ Watery or itchy

____ Swollen

____ Bags or dark circles under eyes

CATEGORY TOTAL: _____

EARS

____ Itchy

____ Ear infections/aches

____ Drainage from ear

____ Ringing

CATEGORY TOTAL: _____

NOSE

____ Stuffy

____ Frequent sinus infections

____ Allergies

____ Excessive mucus formation

CATEGORY TOTAL: _____

MOUTH/THROAT

____ Sore throat, hoarseness, loss of voice

____ Tongue coated white or fuzzy

____ Chronic coughing

____ Canker sores

CATEGORY TOTAL: _____

SKIN

_____ Itchy

_____ Acne

_____ Rashes/hives

_____ Dry

_____ Sweat often

_____ Cold all the time

CATEGORY TOTAL: _____

HEART

_____ Irregular or skipped heartbeat

_____ Rapid heartbeat

_____ Chest pains

CATEGORY TOTAL: _____

LUNGS

_____ Asthma

_____ Difficulty breathing

_____ Shortness of breath

CATEGORY TOTAL: _____

DIGESTIVE TRACT

_____ Bloating

_____ Diarrhea

_____ Constipation

_____ Abdominal pain

_____ Nausea/vomiting

_____ Heartburn

_____ Burping/passing gas

CATEGORY TOTAL: _____

JOINTS/MUSCLES

_____ Joint pains/aching

_____ Stiffness/limitation in movements

_____ Muscle pains/aching

_____ Feeling weak

CATEGORY TOTAL: _____

EATING

_____ Binge eating/drinking

_____ Cravings

_____ Excessive weight gain

_____ Excessive weight loss

_____ Purging

_____ Anorexia/severely decreased caloric intake

_____ Water retention

CATEGORY TOTAL: _____

ENERGY/ACTIVITY

_____ Fatigued, tired all the time

_____ Restless

_____ Hyperactivity

CATEGORY TOTAL: _____

MIND/EMOTIONS

_____ Poor memory, forgetful

_____ Anxious, nervous

_____ Depressed

_____ Irritability, anger

_____ Poor concentration

_____ Slurred speech

CATEGORY TOTAL: _____

Now rate the home and office environmental aspects to your health to add to your total score.

Home/Office Point Scale:
0 = Optimized and good to go!
1 = Working on it
2 = Still have not addressed

AIR

_____ Indoor air filtered

_____ Clean home (dust/wipe/sweep) often

_____ Filters changed timely

_____ Duct work cleaned timely

_____ Open windows to circulate fresh air

CATEGORY TOTAL: _____

WATER

_____ Drinking water filtration system

_____ Shower filtration system

_____ Drink minimum 8 glasses water per day

CATEGORY TOTAL: _____

LIGHT

_____ Outdoor time daily

_____ Red light

_____ Infrared light

CATEGORY TOTAL: _____

MINDSET/STRESS

_____ Time to yourself daily

_____ Reducing stress

_____ Breathing exercises/outdoors/yoga/reading/any relaxation techniques

CATEGORY TOTAL: _____

SLEEP

_____ Go to bed at same time each night

_____ Wake up at same time each morning

_____ Feel rested when awake

_____ No devices 1–2 hours before bed

CATEGORY TOTAL: _____

HOUSEHOLD/HYGIENE

_____ Nontoxic/safer cleaning products

_____ Nontoxic/safer makeup/hygiene products

_____ Organized and clean spaces

CATEGORY TOTAL: _____

GRAND TOTAL: _____

RESULTS

Repeat your Total Toxic Burden score each month to assess your changes and progress.

0 → 10

Minimal Total Toxic Burden. You're doing pretty great with nontoxic and anti-inflammatory living! Awesome work.

11 → 30

Mild Total Toxic Burden. Some room for improvements.

31 → 50

Moderate Total Toxic Burden. Need to make some changes in your environment and lifestyle to reduce toxins before the body declines further. Recommend Maggie Berghoff's Body Reset as well as implementing at least one new lifestyle change from Step Two to reduce toxicities.

51 → 70+

Severe Total Toxic Burden. Recommend Maggie Berghoff's Body Reset to really begin to reduce toxicities and allow the body to heal. In addition, if you are able to, it would be helpful to work with a functional medicine practitioner or coach to help you on this journey.

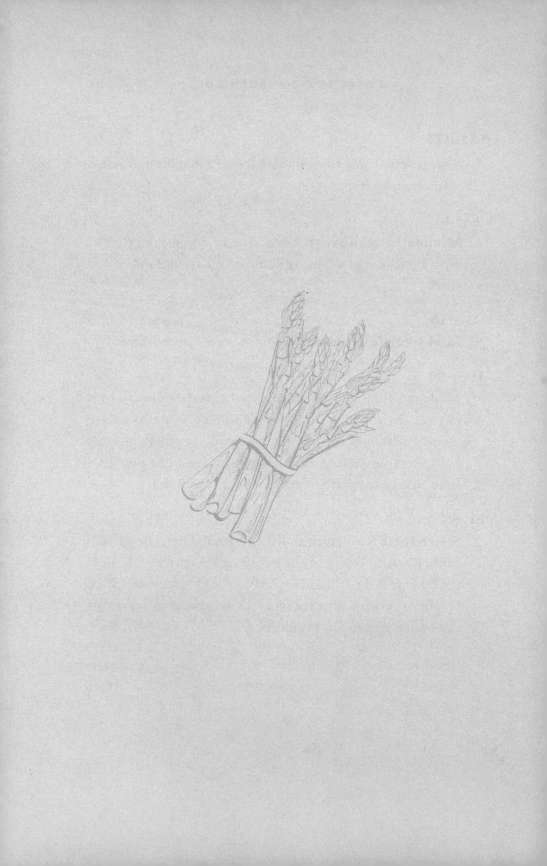

ACKNOWLEDGMENTS

I want to thank my husband, Jimmy, for being so incredibly supportive of all my big dreams. For being the most present and loving father to our three young children.

To my mom, for introducing me to the Institute for Functional Medicine when I was going through my own health challenges, which changed my entire world. To my dad, for instilling strength, work ethic, culture, and adventure in my soul, and for showing us the world.

Thanks to everyone at Park & Fine along with Atria and Simon & Schuster for believing in me and taking a chance on a young and new author. You all are absolutely incredible and it has been a complete honor to be chosen to work with you.

To the leaders in business I look up to. You are inspiring me and paving a path to show me to dream bigger than I would ever imagine.

To my health clients. Every one of you has a permanent place in my heart.

To all the love that poured into this book, the late nights, the early mornings, the typing with one hand while holding a newborn baby with the other. Writing a book has been such an incredible process, I'm so grateful for everyone who helped make this possible.

NOTES

CHAPTER 1: UNDERSTANDING HOW INFLAMMATION WORKS IN YOUR BODY

1 Roy, Sashwati, Debasis Bagchi, and Siba P. Raychaudhuri, *Chronic Inflammation: Molecular Pathophysiology, Nutritional and Therapeutic Interventions* (Oxfordshire: Taylor & Francis, 2012).

2 Chen, L., et al., "Inflammatory Responses and Inflammation-Associated Diseases in Organs," *Oncotarget* 9, no. 6 (2017): 7204–18. https://doi.org /10.18632/oncotarget.23208.

3 Punchard, Neville A., Cliff J. Whelan, and Ian Adcock, "The Journal of Inflammation," *Journal of Inflammation* 1, no. 1 (September 27, 2004): 1. https://doi.org/https://doi.org/10.1186/1476-9255-1-1.

4 Khan, Sal, and David Agus, "Inflammation I Miscellaneous I Health & Medicine I Khan Academy," YouTube, Khan Academy, March 2011. https://www.youtube .com/watch?v=GZ6I3T1RAnQ.

5 Ellulu, Mohammed S., et al., "Obesity and Inflammation: The Linking Mechanism and the Complications," *Archives of Medical Science* 4 (2017): 859. https://doi.org/10.5114/aoms.2016.58928.

6 Punchard, Whelan, and Adcock, "Journal of Inflammation."

7 Roy, Bagchi, and Raychaudhuri, *Chronic Inflammation*.

CHAPTER 3: MUSCLE AND JOINT INFLAMMATION

1 "Arthritis-Related Statistics," Centers for Disease Control and Prevention, July 18, 2018. https://www.cdc.gov/arthritis/data_statistics/arthritis-related-stats.htm.

2 Punchard, Whelan, and Adcock, "Journal of Inflammation."

3 Nettelbladt, Erik G., and Lars K. M. Sundblad, "Protein Patterns in Synovial Fluid and Serum in Rheumatoid Arthritis and Osteoarthritis," *Arthritis & Rheumatology* 2, no. 2 (April 1959): 144–51. https://doi.org/10.1002/1529 -0131(195904)2:2 (144::aid-art1780020206) 3.0.co;2-g.

4 Sokolove, Jeremy, and Christin M. Lepus, "Role of Inflammation in the Pathogenesis of Osteoarthritis: Latest Findings and Interpretations," *Therapeutic Advances in Musculoskeletal Disease* 5, no. 2 (2013): 77–94. https://doi.org /10.1177/1759720x12467868.

5 Gilis, Elisabeth, et al., "The Role of the Microbiome in Gut and Joint Inflammation in Psoriatic Arthritis and Spondyloarthritis," *Journal of Rheumatology* (June 2018). https://doi.org/https://doi.org/10.3899/jrheum.180135.

6 Kadetoff, Diana, et al., "Evidence of Central Inflammation in Fibromyalgia— Increased Cerebrospinal Fluid Interleukin-8 Levels," *Journal of*

Neuroimmunology 242, no. 1–2 (January 2012): 33–38. https://doi.org/https://doi.org/10.1016/j.jneuroim.2011.10.013.

CHAPTER 4: HORMONAL AND THYROID INFLAMMATION

1 Boelaert, Kristien, et al., "Prevalence and Relative Risk of Other Autoimmune Diseases in Subjects with Autoimmune Thyroid Disease," *American Journal of Medicine* 123, no. 2 (2010). https://doi.org/10.1016/j.amjmed.2009.06.030.

2 "Polycystic Ovary Syndrome," womenshealth.gov, April 1, 2019. https://www.womenshealth.gov/a-z-topics/polycystic-ovary-syndrome.

CHAPTER 5: INFLAMMATION FROM SUGAR

1 Saklayen, M. G., "The Global Epidemic of the Metabolic Syndrome," *Current Hypertension Reports* 20, no. 2 (2018): 12. https://doi.org/10.1007/s11906-018-0812-z.

2 Bowman, Shanthy A., et al., "Added Sugars Intake of Americans: What We Eat in America," Food Surveys Research Group Dietary Data Brief No. 18, usda.gov, May 2017. https://www.ars.usda.gov/ARSUserFiles/80400530/pdf/DBrief/18_Added_Sugars_Intake_of_Americans_2013-2014.pdf.

3 "Prediabetes—Your Chance to Prevent Type 2 Diabetes," Centers for Disease Control and Prevention, January 8, 2020. https://www.cdc.gov/diabetes/basics/prediabetes.html.

4 "Diabetes Facts & Figures," International Diabetes Federation—Home, December 2, 2020. https://www.idf.org/aboutdiabetes/what-is-diabetes/facts-figures.html.

CHAPTER 6: PSYCHOLOGICAL STRESS

1 "Facts & Statistics," Anxiety and Depression Association of America, ADAA. Accessed May 12, 2020. https://adaa.org/about adaa/press-room/facts-statistics.

2 Mc Mahon, Brenda, et al., "Seasonal Difference in Brain Serotonin Transporter Binding Predicts Symptom Severity in Patients with Seasonal Affective Disorder," *Brain* 139, no. 5 (2016): 1605–14. https://doi.org/10.1093/brain/aww043.

3 Kemp, Joshua J., James J. Lickel, and Brett J. Deacon, "Effects of a Chemical Imbalance Causal Explanation on Individuals' Perceptions of Their Depressive Symptoms," *Behaviour Research and Therapy* 56 (March 6, 2014): 47–52. https://doi.org/10.1016/j.brat.2014.02.009.

4 Lee, Chieh-Hsin, and Fabrizio Giuliani, "The Role of Inflammation in Depression and Fatigue," *Frontiers in Immunology* 10 (2019). https://doi.org/10.3389/fimmu.2019.01696.

5 Salim, S., G. Chugh, and M. Asghar, "Inflammation in Anxiety," *Advances in Protein Chemistry and Structural Biology* (2012). https://doi.org/10.1016/B978-0-12-398314-5.00001-5.

6 Al-Harbi, K. S., "Treatment-Resistant Depression: Therapeutic Trends, Challenges, and Future Directions," *Patient Preference and Adherence* (2012): 369. https://doi.org/10.2147/ppa.s29716.

7 Felger, Jennifer C., "The Role of Dopamine in Inflammation-Associated Depression: Mechanisms and Therapeutic Implications," *Current Topics in Behavioral Neurosciences* (2016): 199–219. https://doi.org/10.1007/7854_2016_13.

8 Salcedo, Beth, "The Comorbidity of Anxiety and Depression," NAMI. Accessed May 12, 2020. https://www.nami.org/Blogs/NAMI-Blog/January-2018/The -Comorbidity-of-Anxiety-and-Depression.

9 "Biological Link between Stress, Anxiety and Depression Identified," *ScienceDaily*, University of Western Ontario, April 19, 2010. https://www .sciencedaily.com/releases/2010/04/100411143348.htm.

10 Cohen, Sheldon, "How Stress Influences Disease: Study Reveals Inflammation as the Culprit," *ScienceDaily*, Carnegie Mellon University, April 2, 2012. https://www.sciencedaily.com/releases/2012/04/120402162546.htm.

11 "The Brain-Gut Connection," Johns Hopkins Medicine. Accessed May 12, 2020. https://www.hopkinsmedicine.org/health/wellness-and-prevention /the-brain-gut-connection.

CHAPTER 7: DIGESTIVE INFLAMMATION

1 Oz, Helieh S., Sung-Ling Yeh, and Manuela G. Neuman, "Gastrointestinal Inflammation and Repair: Role of Microbiome, Infection, and Nutrition," *Gastroenterology Research and Practice* (2016): 1–3. https://doi.org/10.1155 /2016/6516708.

2 Canavan, C., J. West, and T. Card, "The Epidemiology of Irritable Bowel Syndrome," *Clinical Epidemiology* 6 (2014): 71–80. https://doi.org/10.2147/CLEP.S40245.

3 Mawdsley, J. E., and D. S. Rampton, "Psychological Stress in IBD: New Insights into Pathogenic and Therapeutic Implications," *Gut* 54, no. 10 (January 2005): 1481–91. https://doi.org/10.1136/gut.2005.064261.

CHAPTER 8: ALLERGIES, ASTHMA, AND SKIN INFLAMMATION

1 Salem, Iman, et al., "The Gut Microbiome as a Major Regulator of the Gut-Skin Axis," *Frontiers in Microbiology* 9 (October 2018). https://doi.org/10.3389 /fmicb.2018.01459.

2 O'Neill, C. A., et al., "The Gut-Skin Axis in Health and Disease: A Paradigm with Therapeutic Implications," *Bioessays* 38 (2016): 1167–76. https://doi.org /10.1002/bies.201600008.

3 Bowe, W. P., and A. C. Logan, "Acne Vulgaris, Probiotics and the Gut-Brain-Skin Axis—Back to the Future?" *Gut Pathology* 3, no. 1 (January 31, 2011): 1. https://doi.org/10.1186/1757-4749-3-1.

4 Juhl, Christian, et al., "Dairy Intake and Acne Vulgaris: A Systematic Review and Meta-Analysis of 78,529 Children, Adolescents, and Young Adults," *Nutrients* 10, no. 8 (September 2018): 1049. https://doi.org/10.3390 /nu10081049.

5 Jović, Anamaria, et al., "The Impact of Psychological Stress on Acne," *Acta Dermatovenerologica Croatica (ADC)*, U.S. National Library of Medicine, July 2017. https://www.ncbi.nlm.nih.gov/pubmed/28871928.

6 Lee, So Yeon, et al., "Microbiome in the Gut-Skin Axis in Atopic Dermatitis," *Allergy, Asthma & Immunology Research*, Korean Academy of Asthma, Allergy and Clinical Immunology; Korean Academy of Pediatric Allergy and Respiratory Disease, July 2018. https://www.ncbi.nlm.nih.gov/pmc/articles/PMC6021588/.

7 Fraser, Kathleen, and Lynne Robertson, "Chronic Urticaria and Autoimmunity," *Skin Therapy Letter*, U.S. National Library of Medicine, 2013. https://www.ncbi .nlm.nih.gov/pubmed/24305753.

CHAPTER 9: MINDSET AND MINDFULNESS

1 "Joe Dispenza on the Power of Thought Alone to Heal," *Natural Awakenings*, July 31, 2015. https://www.naturalawakenings.com/2015/07/31/224946 /joe-dispenza-on-the-power-of-thought-alone-to-heal.

2 Dispenza, Joe, *Breaking the Habit of Being Yourself: How to Lose Your Mind and Create a New One* (Carlsbad, CA: Hay House, 2016).

3 Avey, Holly, et al., "Health Care Providers' Training, Perceptions, and Practices Regarding Stress and Health Outcomes," *Journal of the National Medical Association* (2003): 833–45. https://www.ncbi.nlm.nih.gov/pmc/articles /PMC2594476/pdf/jnma00313-0070.pdf.

4 Roser, Max, and Esteban Ortiz-Ospina, "Literacy," *Our World in Data*, September 20, 2018. https://ourworldindata.org/literacy.

CHAPTER 10: DETOXIFY AND OPTIMIZE YOUR HOME AND OFFICE ENVIRONMENT

1 "Health Hazards in Common Home Products," Northwest Natural Medicine, November 25, 2015. https://nwnaturalmedicine.com/health-hazards-in-common -home-products/.

2 Sholl, Jessie, et al., "8 Hidden Toxins: What's Lurking in Your Cleaning Products?" *Experience Life*, February 14, 2020. https://experiencelife.com/article /8-hidden-toxins-whats-lurking-in-your-cleaning-products/.

3 "Detoxification—Heavy Metals," Natural Health Improvement Center. Accessed May 12, 2020. https://www.nhicwestmi.com/detoxification-heavy-metals.

4 https://www.epa.gov/mercury/how-people-are-exposed-mercury.

5 https://www.epa.gov/mercury/basic-information-about-mercury#airemissions.

6 https://www.epa.gov/sites/production/files/2018-07/documents/nei2014v2_tsd _05jul2018.pdf.

7 https://www.epa.gov/lead/protect-your-family-exposures-lead#water.

8 https://www.epa.gov/lead/lead-outdoor-air.

9 https://www.epa.gov/lead/protect-your-family-exposures-lead#soil.

10 https://www.epa.gov/sites/production/files/2016-09/documents/cadmium -compounds.pdf.

11 https://www.epa.gov/sites/production/files/2014-03/documents/arsenic_toxfaqs _3v.pdf.

12 http://www.idph.state.il.us/envhealth/factsheets/zinc.htm.

13 https://www.atsdr.cdc.gov/phs/phs.asp?id=243&tid=44

14 https://www.atsdr.cdc.gov/phs/phs.asp?id=307&tid=49

15 https://www.atsdr.cdc.gov/phs/phs.asp?id=1076&tid=34

16 https://www.epa.gov/sites/production/files/2016-09/documents/phosphorus.pdf

17 University of Wisconsin Hospitals and Clinics Authority, "The Benefits of Drinking Water for Your Skin," UW Health. Accessed May 12, 2020. https://www.uwhealth.org/madison-plastic-surgery/the-benefits-of-drinking-water-for-your-skin/26334.

18 "Health Benefits of Matcha Tea," Matcha Source. Accessed May 12, 2020. https://matchasource.com/health-benefits-of-matcha-tea/.

19 https://www.epa.gov/sites/production/files/2016-03/documents/occtmarch2016.pdf.

20 Fedinick, K. P., et al., "Threats on Tap: Widespread Violations Highlight Need for Investment in Water Infrastructure and Protections," *Natural Resources Defense Council* (2017): 1–26. https://www.nrdc.org/resources/threats-tap-widespread-violations-water-infrastructure.

21 https://www.ncbi.nlm.nih.gov/pubmed/21527855.

22 Blume, C., C. Garbazza, and M. Spitschan, "Effects of Light on Human Circadian Rhythms, Sleep and Mood," *Somnologie (Berl)* 23, no. 3 (2019): 147–56. doi:10.1007/s11818-019-00215-x.

23 Potter G. D., et al., "Circadian Rhythm and Sleep Disruption: Causes, Metabolic Consequences, and Countermeasures," *Endocrine Review* 37, no. 6 (2016): 584–608. doi:10.1210/er.2016-1083.

24 https://www.health.harvard.edu/staying-healthy/blue-light-has-a-dark-side.

25 Markwald, R. R., et al., "Impact of Insufficient Sleep on Total Daily Energy Expenditure, Food Intake, and Weight Gain," *Proceedings of the National Academy of Sciences of the United States of America* 110, no. 14 (2013): 5695–700. https://doi.org/10.1073/pnas.1216951110.

26 Chevalier, G., G. Melvin, and T. Barsotti, "One-Hour Contact with the Earth's Surface (Grounding) Improves Inflammation and Blood Flow—A Randomized, Double-Blind, Pilot Study," *Health* 7, no. 8 (2015): 1022–59. doi: 10.4236/health.2015.78119.

27 "The Never List," Beautycounter. Accessed May 12, 2020. https://www.beautycounter.com/the-never-list.

28 "Cosmetics and Your Health," National Institute of Environmental Health Sciences, U.S. Department of Health and Human Services. Accessed May 12, 2020. https://www.niehs.nih.gov/health/topics/agents/cosmetics/index.cfm.

29 "Triclosan," Government of Canada, Health, August 23, 2019. https://www.canada.ca/en/health-canada/services/chemicals-product-safety/triclosan.html.

CHAPTER 11: SUPERCHARGE YOUR IMMUNE SYSTEM

1 Harvard Health Publishing, "What You Should Know about Magnesium," *Healthbeat*. Accessed May 12, 2020. https://www.health.harvard.edu/staying-healthy/what-you-should-know-about-magnesium2.

2 Clear, James, *Atomic Habits: Tiny Changes, Remarkable Results—An Easy & Proven Way to Build Good Habits & Break Bad Ones* (New York: Avery, 2018).

CHAPTER 12: EXERCISE AND MOVEMENT

1 Warburton, D. E., C. W. Nicol, and S. S. Bredin, "Health Benefits of Physical Activity: The Evidence," *Canadian Medical Association Journal* 174, no. 6 (2006): 801–9. https://doi.org/10.1503/cmaj.051351.1.

2 Takács, Johanna, "Regular Physical Activity and Mental Health. The Role of Exercise in the Prevention of, and Intervention in Depressive Disorders," *Psychiatria Hungarica: A Magyar Pszichiatriai Tarsasag tudomanyos folyoirata*, U.S. National Library of Medicine, 2014. https://www.ncbi.nlm.nih.gov/pubmed/25569828.

3 Teixeira, Pedro J., et al., "Exercise, Physical Activity, and Self-Determination Theory: A Systematic Review," *International Journal of Behavioral Nutrition and Physical Activity*, BioMed Central, June 22, 2012. https://www.ncbi.nlm.nih.gov/pmc/articles/PMC3441783/.

4 Panton, Lynn B., and Ashley L. Artese, "Types of Exercise: Flexibility, Strength, Endurance, Balance," SpringerLink, Springer, Cham, January 1, 1970. https://link.springer.com/chapter/10.1007/978-3-319-16095-5_4.

5 Lumsden, Joanne, Lynden K. Miles, and C. Neil Macrae, "Sync or Sink? Interpersonal Synchrony Impacts Self-Esteem," *Frontiers in Psychology* 5 (2014). https://doi.org/10.3389/fpsyg.2014.01064.

6 Woods, Jeffrey A., et al., "Exercise, Inflammation and Aging," *Aging and Disease*, JKL International LLC, February 2012. https://www.ncbi.nlm.nih.gov/pmc/articles/PMC3320801/.

7 Anderson, Elizabeth, and Geetha Shivakumar, "Effects of Exercise and Physical Activity on Anxiety," *Frontiers in Psychiatry* 4 (2013). https://doi.org/10.3389/fpsyt.2013.00027.

8 Payne, Peter, and Mardi A. Crane-Godreau, "Meditative Movement for Depression and Anxiety," *Frontiers in Psychiatry*, Frontiers Media S.A., July 24, 2013. https://www.ncbi.nlm.nih.gov/pubmed/23898306.

CHAPTER 13: YOUR ANTI-INFLAMMATORY PANTRY AND FRIDGE

1 Hari, Vani, "Ingredients to Avoid in Processed Food," Food Babe. Accessed May 12, 2020. https://foodbabe.com/ingredients-to-avoid/.

2 Ericson, John. "75% of Americans May Suffer from Chronic Dehydration, According to Doctors." Medical Daily, July 4, 2013. https://www.medicaldaily.com/75-americans-may-suffer-chronic-dehydration-according-doctors-247393.

INDEX

ABOUT THE AUTHOR

MAGGIE BERGHOFF, FNP-C, is an expert health and wellness consultant and entrepreneur. She is the founder and CEO of Celproceo, a revolutionary health and wellness agency that empowers and encourages individuals to transform into stronger and healthier versions of themselves through innovative and personalized programs. Maggie is trusted by CEOs, top organizations, celebrities, and professional athletes to elevate personal performance through cocreated practices rooted in functional and integrative medicine. A global wellness expert, Maggie has been featured in *Forbes*, *USA TODAY*, *Business Insider*, *Oxygen Magazine*, *Glamour*, and many more. Maggie is also a mother to three young children. Visit maggieberghoff.com and follow her on Instagram @Maggie_Berghoff.